Cong
A 4 U.

With my Book
inspire you in your
Hot ... January

[signature]

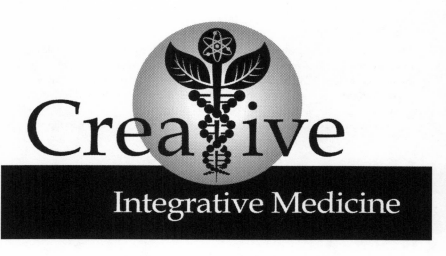

Crea🜨ive
Integrative Medicine

A Medical Doctor's Journey
toward a New Vision for Health Care

Dr. Paul Drouin, M.D.

BALBOA.
PRESS
A DIVISION OF HAY HOUSE

Balboa Press books may be ordered through booksellers or by contacting:

Balboa Press
A Division of Hay House
1663 Liberty Drive
Bloomington, IN 47403
www.balboapress.com
1 (877) 407-4847

Because of the dynamic nature of the Internet, any web addresses or links contained in this book may have changed since publication and may no longer be valid. The views expressed in this work are solely those of the author and do not necessarily reflect the views of the publisher, and the publisher hereby disclaims any responsibility for them.

The author of this book does not dispense medical advice or prescribe the use of any technique as a form of treatment for physical, emotional, or medical problems without the advice of a physician, either directly or indirectly. The intent of the author is only to offer information of a general nature to help you in your quest for emotional and spiritual well-being. In the event you use any of the information in this book for yourself, which is your constitutional right, the author and the publisher assume no responsibility for your actions.

Any people depicted in stock imagery provided by Thinkstock are models, and such images are being used for illustrative purposes only.
Certain stock imagery © Thinkstock.

Printed in the United States of America.

ISBN: 978-1-4525-1843-5 (sc)
ISBN: 978-1-4525-1845-9 (hc)
ISBN: 978-1-4525-1844-2 (e)

Library of Congress Control Number: 2014912459

Balboa Press rev. date: 08/01/2014

To my brother, who is the reason for this book.

To my mother, who taught me love and compassion.

And to our family doctor, who showed me how to go beyond the usual path …

Contents

Foreword

It is a pleasure for me to write the foreword for this book because it is complementary to my own work toward developing an integrative framework for the practice of medicine. I have been approaching the subject of integrating alternative and conventional medical practices into one integrative whole using an integrative paradigm of science that quantum physics bestows upon us. But I am not a healer; I have no experience in practicing medicine with actual patients. So I am super-delighted that now somebody of the caliber of Dr. Paul Drouin, who is a trained practitioner of both conventional medicine and of some of the alternative medicine practices, has joined the task of bringing the quantum point of view toward integrating the disparate medicine practices that he participates in under one umbrella of a truly integrative medicine. And he does this from a practitioner's point of view. This is a most significant development.

That the quantum worldview would revolutionize medicine is now a three-decades-old idea. In the first phase, the physician Larry Dossey emphasized the importance of quantum nonlocality (signal-less communication) that subsequently found verification in the distant prayer-healing experiments. And the physician Deepak Chopra introduced quantum leaps of quantum healing to explain the many known cases of spontaneous healing of cancer without medical intervention.

In the second phase, I developed a theoretical framework for integrative medicine using the principles of quantum physics that call for the primacy of consciousness as the fabric of reality.

Dr. Drouin's book signals the beginning of a third phase: the application of the quantum theory of integrative medicine to actual cases of healing complete with documented case histories. But that is just one important aspect of the book. Paul Drouin's own take of how integrative medicine, integrating one or more alternative medicine practices with conventional allopathy, actually works is also wonderfully enlightening. What is also striking is that there is much original insight here that only the actual practice of quantum integrative medicine could have revealed.

But Dr. Drouin, not being a quantum physicist, avoids an in-depth introductory discussion of the quantum worldview and how it gives us a basis for a quantum integrative medicine. However, to you, dear reader, such a discussion may be useful before delving into the delights of this book. Hence this foreword from a quantum physicist will now aim to fill this omission.

The Quantum Worldview as a Basis for a Quantum Integrative Medicine

Quantum physics says, contradicting the "hard" scientists like our conventional medicine practitioners from the get go, objects are waves of possibility. They reside outside of space and time in a domain—call it the domain of potentiality—experimentally characterized by instant signal-less communication or nonlocality. What converts these waves of possibility to the particles of actuality in space and time when we observe them? A little analysis reveals this: first, if you think consciousness is brain phenomenon, you get unsolvable paradoxes. Quantum physics implies that consciousness is the ground of being in which the many-facetted possibility objects reside. Second, it is the causal act of choice by consciousness that collapses the waves of possibility into particles of actuality converting them from a many-facetted object to a one-facetted one.

But sensing material objects is just one of our experiences. We have other experiences. We have feeling. What do we feel? Next time you have a strong emotion, try to feel it viscerally, in your body. Especially, put your attention along your spine. You will feel movements—vital energy that Indians call *prana* and the Chinese call *chi*. And, of course, we think. We think story lines, but at a subtler level, we think meaning. At an even subtler level, we intuit. These experiences of intuitions give us the contexts of our most profound meanings. Plato called the objects of experience in intuition archetypes.

Scientists until very recently have recognized, in agreement with Plato, that archetypes are timeless, they are not material. Even today, many scientists agree that science's pursuit of universal scientific laws is a pursuit of the timeless archetype of truth. However, although ordinary people would agree that we think with our mind, many scientists think that mind is made of brain. Similarly, biologists almost unanimously deny the existence of vital energy as anything nonphysical.

But fortunately, recent work by the biologist Rupert Sheldrake has shown that biology needs nonphysical entities that he calls morphogenetic fields to explain how biological form is made. We can easily realize that what we feel as vital energy is the movement of morphogenetic fields since the energies that we feel, we feel at "chakra" points along the spine, and always close to where one or another of the important organs (biological forms) of the body are found. Further realize that the organs are physical representations of the morphogenetic fields that now you should think as blueprints of organs.

And the philosopher John Searle and the physicist Roger Penrose have demonstrated that computers cannot process meaning. Since even according to the neurophysiologists, brain is a sort of a computer, the idea that mind is brain is ruled out. Mind is also nonphysical.

But there is a problem with this kind of thinking. Scientists call this kind of thinking dualism, and the problem is how a physical world can interact with a nonphysical world. These scientists think with Newtonian physics according to which all interactions require signals through space and time and involve exchange of energy. Since energy of the physical world alone is always a constant, dualism seems to be incompatible with science.

But only until you recognize quantum physics and the quantum worldview. Recall that the nonlocal domain of potentiality is consciousness, and imagine that in it are embodied four different worlds of four different kinds of possibility objects from which our four different kinds of experiences originate. When we sense, we are choosing from the potentiality of the physical and collapsing material objects in space and time. When we choose from the vital world from the possibilities of the morphogenetic blueprints, it is the changes in the latter that we experience as the feeling of vital energy. When we choose from the meaning possibilities of the mind, we experience thinking. And finally, choosing from the archetypal possibility world gives us the experience of intuition.

What mediates the interaction between the disparate worlds? No signals are needed; nonlocal consciousness mediates. This solution is crucial for integrating conventional material science of medicine with nonmaterial or subtle sciences of medicine that we call alternative medicine.

We need one more idea. In the physical world, we have structure. This is because in the physical, micro elementary particles make up macro stuff—chairs, the human brain. But in the subtle worlds, there is micro macro division. Three consequences: first, macrophysical loses most of its quantum potency and is approximately Newtonian—deterministic, not much play of possibilities there. So your choice and my choice tend to be virtually the same when we look at a particular object, and we can build a consensus that we are seeing the same thing at the same place and that the object is outside of us. Subtle objects—feeling, thinking, and intuition—they are quantum all the way; you and I cannot choose the same experience ordinarily, making the experiences private and internal.

Second, the fixity of the macrophysical world gives us reference points for our bodies. Most importantly, it also enables the physical to make representations, "software," of the subtle hardware.

Third, the way these representations are built as we grow up gives us patterns of conditioning that give us functional individuality. Our individual mind and individual vital body are the results of the conditioning—they are functional bodies, not structural.

Now the conceptual basis of quantum integrative medicine can be stated. First, we have three individual bodies—physical, vital, and mental. Disease can occur due to the lack of balance and harmony in any and all of these bodies. And healing, likewise, would consist of not only restoring the structural malfunction of the physical but also functional malfunction of the vital and mental, if any.

Second, in truth, although the archetypal (that elsewhere I refer to as supramental) world is not directly represented in the physical at this stage of our evolution, we can think of that entire world as a common body that we all share.

And finally, even consciousness as a whole can be thought of as a limitless body for all of us to share. When we identify with this body, we experience wholeness that makes us happy. You can think of it as a happiness body.

So integrative medicine: five different bodies, five kinds of disease depending on where the root of the disease lies, and five kinds of healing beginning with the healing of the root cause. To repeat, conventional medicine is about physical body disease and healing. Vital body medicine is about healing vital body malfunction, malfunction of the vital correlates (the morphogenetic blueprints) of the organs, causing malfunctions of the physical organs. Examples are: Indian Ayurveda, Traditional Chinese medicine, and homeopathy. Mind-body medicine is about healing malfunctions of the mental body that cause malfunction of the vital and the physical. And so forth.

Creativity

Dr. Paul Drouin's genius takes us one step further. He refers to quantum integrative medicine as creative integrative medicine, in this way injecting the important idea that quantum creativity can be part and parcel of all integrative medicine practice involving a subtle body. Why restrict quantum healing to chance spontaneity? Why not use the creative process to precipitate quantum healing whenever needed?

Dr. Drouin's creativity in the book does not end there, of course. Previously I mentioned originality. You will especially enjoy his presentation of Taoist medicine and also his idea of using measurements of blood as a diagnostic tool of integrative medicine.

I should note that this book developed not only from Drouin's experiences as a physician of both conventional and alternative medicine, but also from his dogged perseverance in developing an institution of teaching integrative medicine. He is the founder of Quantum University, which has trained hundreds of students in this creative quantum integrative medicine.

I will end with a personal anecdote. You will find Dr. Drouin himself talking about his French accent in the book and how that made it difficult for him to teach in English-speaking America. When I first heard him in a classroom situation, he was talking about the creative ah-ha experience, ah-ha denoting the surprise of a quantum leap of course. Unfortunately his French accent made him sound like he was speaking of "ha-ha" experience. Initially I was amused, ha-ha amused. But then a very sweet thought came over me as I looked at him. He *was* in the middle of what is called a flow experience where instead of the ah-ha surprise, you feel joyful (ha-ha?) flow. This man really loves interacting with his students, I thought as I became a part of the same flow.

When I read the book, this was again my experience—flow; I became a part of the author's joy of presenting his ideas and his life to teach something that he believes in. I hope your experience will be similar.

I have no doubt that this book will be celebrated by all practitioners of alternative medicine. For the hard-core conventional medical practitioner, I will say this: quantum physics has passed the test of time for almost a hundred years and its message is now clear and loud. Reality is made of consciousness. Newtonian machine medicine has to give way to quantum creative integrative medicine for the living and the conscious. My book, *The Quantum Doctor*, has given you the theory. This book will give you data that quantum integrative medicine works and it can be extended to make it ever more powerful. Read the book. In the least, it will help to open your mind.

– Amit Goswami, PhD
Quantum physicist and the author of *The Self-aware Universe, The Quantum Doctor*, and *Quantum Creativity: Think Quantum, Be Creative.*

Note from Author

No one knows the price we are paying for an incomplete medical education.

In writing this book, I would like to bring to the reader an awareness of a new vision for health care. Today, thousands of explorers and pioneers in the healing profession are coming to the same conclusion: that it is necessary for us to redefine a new foundation for the future of modern medicine. Through my own awakening as a medical doctor, I too have come to this realization, which has led me to creative integrative medicine.

Humbly, I would now like to share my own experiences as a medical and integrative clinician, healer, and educator on a subject that has been my passion for most of my life: medicine.

Preface

Science defines the premise upon which our understanding of reality is based. Traditionalists have declared that conventional Western medicine is the only scientific medicine. The current medical system is based upon a materialistic model incorporating Darwinist theories of evolution, Newtonian physics, chemistry, physical (elementary particle level) anatomy, and physiology. However, through explorations and observations of the behavior of particles at the subatomic level, science has continued to evolve. Fifty years ago, quantum physics emerged as a new scientific standard and model for our understanding of reality. It has revolutionized our society on many levels, sparking discussion of science versus spirituality/consciousness and transforming the core of our society.

It is now time to redefine a form of medicine based on the new scientific model of understanding of the universe according to quantum physics—a creative integrative medicine. Doing so will be the key to solving the current health-care crisis, and it will lead to a new vision of integrative health care based not on disease but on the full potential of the individual. Our understanding of the human body will expand to include the body's subtle energy systems and the mental and emotional connections to the physical body. How the mind works can be explored from a nondualistic viewpoint, compared to the dualistic philosophy used today. It will open the door to creative new approaches to healing that have the opportunity to solve problems still unresolved by conventional medicine, specifically in the areas of chronic and degenerative diseases.

My journey as a doctor in Western medicine began over forty years ago in Québec, Canada. While in medical school and in the early days of my own family practice, I began to see the limitations of conventional Western medical approaches, not only in the areas of diagnosis and treatment of patients but also in how a patient was viewed and how the greater issues of pain and suffering were left unaddressed. Deep within, I felt there was a better way. This led me on an ongoing journey of discovery as I explored alternative medical traditions, such as Ayurvedic medicine, Taoist Chinese medicine and acupuncture, homeopathy, auriculotherapy, naturopathy, mind-body medicine, emerging diagnostics techniques in dark field microscopy, and Kirlian photography. As I learned new modalities, I incorporated them into my family practice alongside conventional medical procedures, creating my own form of integrative family medicine practice. During this process, I began formulating a holistic view of patients and looked at their potential for wellness, rather than focusing solely on their physical symptoms of disease.

Patients were very responsive to this approach, and I grew a successful family practice, primarily through referrals. I was able to treat a large number of patients who had not found satisfactory assistance within the conventional Western health-care system. However, as peers began to learn of my work with complementary and alternative medicine, my approach was criticized as being nonscientific and not something that was taught in medical school.

Although many studies have been performed to assess the benefits of these alternative modalities, the conventional medical system and medical schools have been slow to adopt, integrate, and train doctors in these alternative therapies and approaches to healing. The primary argument that has been given is the lack of scientific basis or lack of scientific explanation for how or why these modalities work.

In my own practice, I saw how effective an integrative approach to medicine could be, and I began searching for the scientific proof of why these modalities worked. I discovered the explanation through the science of physics, which I believe can serve as the new scientific foundation for a truly integrative medicine that combines both Western and alternative medicine systems and traditions based on a platform of understanding of the new scientific reality as defined by quantum physics. Quantum physicist Amit Goswami, PhD, has already laid out the theoretical foundation for this approach in his book *The Quantum Doctor, a physicist's guide to health and healing* (2004).

The curriculum I've developed for holistic, natural, and integrative medicine at Quantum University already incorporates this paradigm of understanding reality based on the science of quantum physics and how it can be applied to healing. It is my hope that other medical universities will soon follow.

This book is a story about my own journey as a medical doctor toward creative integrative medicine. It is about my passion to promote changes in the health-care systems and medical schools that will lead to a greater understanding of the true nature of the human being and assist us in reaching our greatest potential through healing on all levels.

Acknowledgments

Before embarking upon this extraordinary journey toward a new vision for health care, I would like express my gratitude to everyone who has been with me on my path, guiding or supporting me in a process which is continuously evolving.

God is the major reference for many of us, so surely He should be at the top of this list. But there are also special human beings in one's life who are significant determinants, and it's impossible to imagine how one's reality could have manifested without them being major actors in the play. As you will read in this book, the illness my youngest brother, Jacques, suffered and the unconditional love of my mother, Valerie, caring for him served as the trigger for my entire journey. Our family doctor, Dr. Victor Cloutier, through his total dedication to my brother and the whole family, has certainly been an inspiration for this book and a model for my entire professional career. I am very pleased to finally be able to acknowledge his deep influence on my life.

I would especially like to thank my son, Alexi, who is also my best friend and a partner who has helped make the realization of Quantum University possible. We came to the United States together in the year 2000, when the university was only a concept. At that time, he was in college with the dream of becoming an actor, like many others his age. He later graduated in Los Angeles as a film and video producer and has since become the mastermind of all the complexities of establishing an online university organization, incorporating the latest features of modern technology.

His dedication and creativity have allowed the International University of Integrative Medicine (IQUIM) to become not only a reality but also an *American dream* story. I remember in the beginning, when we were participating in naturopathic conventions and looking at other colleges and natural medicine universities, we were very impressed and in some ways intimidated. Since then, we have made our own claim for recognition and today are seen as leaders in this field. We could certainly write another book about our adventures together and—who knows?—perhaps make another *American dream* story movie. But this one will feature two French Canadians who came to America at the beginning of the century to try to make a difference in health-care education.

I also want to thank my daughter, Estelle, who has been for me an inspiration as the mother of two sons, Isaiah and Thomas, painting artist, and yoga teacher. My quest to find other means of healing was recently challenged again when just over a year ago she gave birth three months prematurely to Thomas Knox. Her unconditional love and commitment to life have shown me the truest expression of what should be at the heart of medicine.

MariaLuz Ramos also played a pivotal role in the establishment of the first years of the Quantum University. Without her dedication and help, the University would not have been born. I would also like to recognize the crucial contributions of all those who have participated in the realization of Quantum University: Michelle Halvorson, Victoria Mathieu, Dr. Andrea Mills, Dr. Charlene Reeves, and Alvan and Denise Pepito. More recently others have added their skills and competence to complement the team: Paul Pono Martin, Mark Valenti, Elizabeth Buck, Dr. Patricia Knox, and Mike O'Leary. I appreciate your contributions.

Special thanks to Adriane Holliman who is developing our new holistic medical assistant program, with the aid of Francine Rodgers and Vedas Burkeen. Bravo for your good work.

I have also to acknowledge the work of Patricia Tello and Dr. Maria Eugenia Sanchez for the Spanish translation of our programs.

There are many others to thank who have supported the realization of this book. Thank you to Cara Waters for her invaluable assistance with the language of Shakespeare in editing this book. I have also to mention my sincere appreciation to Susan Murray, who has patiently reviewed the manuscript and prepared it for the publisher.

I would like to express my deep appreciation for Dr. Amit Goswami, who has been not only a great inspiration for this book but has also been a significant contributor to the curriculum of the university. Many others are part of this great adventure at Quantum University and have influenced its curriculum. To Dr. Joe Dispenza, Dr. Jeffrey Fannin, Dr. Bruce Lipton, Dr. Yury Kronn, Dr. Patrick Porter, Dr. Cynthia J. Porter, Dr. Gaetan Chevalier, Dr. Faith Nelson, Dr. Debrah Zepf, Dr. Terry Oleson, Lynne McTaggart, and many others, I am pleased to say, "Thank you. I am grateful."

I am also deeply grateful to my dear students. They are the ones who carry this mission around the world. Without their support and encouragement, we would never have been able to manifest our vision for creative integrative medicine. They are making our dream a reality.

Finally, I would like to thank Hay House for this amazing opportunity to participate in and receive an award for this book in the Writing from Your Soul contest. Thanks to you, this book's publication is now being facilitated through the Balboa Press Inspire Publishing Package.

Introduction

A Family Tragedy

My path toward becoming a medical doctor was sparked by a deeply personal and traumatic life experience. As a teenager living in rural Québec, Canada, in 1966, I watched as my own brother suffered from ongoing headaches and my mother took him from doctor to doctor for a year without obtaining a proper diagnosis of his symptoms. After traveling to Québec City to see several specialists, they all concluded that his condition was psychosomatic.

Once a patient is tagged with a diagnosis, a family doctor will rarely contest or question the finding. However, our family doctor did, and I was impressed by that. To this day, I see him as a hero in that regard. Unsatisfied with the outcome from my brother's visits to the specialists, he took it upon himself to arrange for my brother to travel to Boston, Massachusetts, to seek further medical assistance. There, he was finally diagnosed with osteosarcoma of the skull—a rare, untreatable form of bone cancer. With no treatment options or hope for recovery, he returned home and our family watched helplessly as he progressively declined and eventually died.

I had a deep feeling of powerlessness during this time—without the knowledge, resources, or solution to be able to help him. It was as a witness to this traumatic family event that I began my quest, an existential search for answers to the questions: Why pain? Why suffering? Why was their view so fatalistic, and why could they do nothing to help my brother? It was then that I decided I would go to medical school, determined to investigate and search for answers to these questions as well as to explore other approaches to cancer and chronic diseases.

Medical School

As a medical student from 1970–1976, I became disappointed with the symptomatic, mechanistic approach to suffering and disease. Prescription for pharmaceuticals (one of the largest costs for the health-care system, often with side effects) was the symptomatic treatment. There was no real cure offered for chronic diseases. I found myself in a dichotomy in medical school. I felt I didn't belong there. What I was being taught did not satisfy my expectations of what it was I had hoped to learn. The diagnostic approaches being used were missing some important aspects I felt needed to be explored. Having had the opportunity to review my brother's old medical files, I wondered how the initial specialists all got it so wrong: why were they not able to diagnose him properly? I saw the fragility of the evaluation process.

I realized that I couldn't find the answers about suffering, pain, and disease in conventional medicine. While in medical school, I began to explore the concepts of other models of medicine. I wanted to understand the depth of the whole issue of suffering and how it relates to the mind and how the mind and body are related to each other. Already in the 1970s, literature had been written on consciousness, relaxation, yoga, and psychosomatics. Before medical school, I had already been exposed to the work of Carl Jung and had delved even further into my explorations of mind, spirit, and the depth of understanding of the soul. His teachings also introduced me to the movement of consciousness in psychology. Jung became the subject of my thesis, and at one point, I considered pursuing a career as a psychiatrist.

I studied biology and evolutionary theory. Finding Darwin's approach to evolution unsatisfactory, I pursued my own personal research in this area. In my college years, I became familiar with the French Jesuit priest, philosopher, and paleontologist Pierre Teilhard de Chardin and his writings on evolutionary concepts. At the time, I realized the link with the emergent literature on consciousness. When I was exposed to scientific literature written on transcendental meditation, I deepened my own practice of meditation and yoga.

In the regular medical school curriculum, I felt there was no real attempt to understand the core of things. In 1975, I obtained my LMCC medical license from the College of Physicians and Surgeons of Québec, Canada. By the time I graduated with a certificate in family medicine in 1976, I had more questions than answers.

As a young doctor, I decided to begin a family practice in rural Québec, living and breathing the standard model of medicine I had learned at school. I traveled to northern Canada to help serve the Inuit and Native Indian populations. It was an exciting time to be a doctor in Canada, with the advent of universal health care and the Centre Locale Service Communautaire (CLSC) system in Québec. I was even one of the founders at the beginning of the creation of these centers. I thought that social medicine was a positive change because everyone would have access to health care. I argued with the older doctors, who were accustomed to their private practices, that this was a better way. Under the new system, doctors were paid by salary or by government health insurance.

Exploring the Mind-Body Connection in Switzerland

After two years of conventional medical practice, I began to ask, "Is there a way to do medicine differently?" I took a sabbatical year from my practice and traveled to Switzerland to study in a specialized one-year training program with a group of physicians from around the world. While there, I was introduced to Ayurvedic medicine, one of the world's oldest systems of medicine, which originated in India.

As a group of physicians, we explored the connection between mind and body, psychosomatic disease and different levels of consciousness. We researched and scientifically studied the effects of consistent meditation practices and relaxation techniques on brain waves and brain physiology. Our experiences were later documented in the article "Méditation Transcendantale Revue de la Littérature Scientifique" in *Le Médecin de Québec* (Blicher 1980).

This article marked the beginning of the study of the physiology of altered states of consciousness, which had been introduced a few years earlier by Fritjof Capra in his book *The Tao of Physics*. In it, he explored "this relationship between the concepts of modern physics and the basic ideas in the philosophical and religious traditions of the Far East" regarding our perception of reality (Capra 1975). We were trying to find the bridge between consciousness and science. Today, quantum physics provides this bridge.

Studies in Alternative Medicine: Developing an Integrative Medical Practice

My year in Switzerland, with all that I learned and experienced, established within me the seed of a vision. As I returned to Québec and took a job as an emergency doctor, I realized I was experiencing an increased level of mental sharpness and coordination as I worked, which I attributed to the meditation practices I had participated in while overseas. When I returned, I had an inner vision with no way of expressing it in the environment in which I was working. I was frustrated by seeing patients who came to the hospital without a reason for emergency. I thought that in these cases, educating the people on the impact of lifestyle and food would be a better approach than just treating them, but that was not happening there. There was a gap between the vision I had and the reality of what I was doing. My reality didn't fit with what I wanted to do. I found myself in an uncomfortable place.

After six months in emergency medicine, I decided to return to family practice. Over the next five years, as I faced the wide variety of challenges experienced by most general family practitioners, I saw limitations of what I was doing with standard medical approaches. Gradually, based on the foundation of what I had learned in Switzerland, I began exploring more complementary alternative medicine options and integrating them into my practice.

In wintertime, children were often brought to me with the common complaints of recurrent otitis and chronic infections, and I prescribed the traditional regimen of antibiotics. After two to three years, as the same children would return to me with the same issues and I prescribed yet another round of antibiotics, I began to question their repetitive use. This led me to enroll in a five-year training program in homeopathy offered through the Association de Medicine Holistique du Québec. Dr. Jacques Jouani (University of Lyon), Dr. Denis Démarque (University of Bordeaux), and Dr. Jean-Bernard Crapan (University of Dijon) traveled from France to Québec to teach the program. I also did complementary studies in homeopathy with the Mosane School of Belgium and with Dr. Jean-Pierre Muyard at the Natural Therapeutics Institute in Québec, Canada. By the mid-1980s I was board certified in homeopathy and began to incorporate homeopathy in treating children with chronic infections, such as chronic fatigue syndrome and allergies, with good results.

I continued to travel throughout Europe, Canada, and the United States to learn more about alternative medicine. From 1986 to 1990, I studied acupuncture through the College of Physicians and Surgeons of Québec, in collaboration with the Acupuncture Foundation of Canada, and subsequently became the second Québec doctor to be licensed in acupuncture. Over this same period, I studied and became certified in the Cyriax techniques of orthopedic medicine, as taught by the British Society of Orthopedic Medicine. I went to Florida to study nutrition at the Hippocrates Health Institute, where I learned about live foods, sprouting, and the use of diet in treating disease.

To further supplement my knowledge of acupuncture, I embarked on the study of auriculotherapy based on the principles of auriculomedicine, founded by Dr. Paul Nogier. In auriculomedicine, the principle is that certain zones or points on the external ear can be mapped to related body organs and systems. Stimulating a specific point on the ear causes a reflex action in the corresponding area of the body. I began to integrate auriculotherapy techniques into my practice and found them particularly successful in the treatment of back and cervical pain.

In order to be able to perform more quantitative measurements at acupuncture points, I purchased a first-generation micro current device and a Vega Electro-Dermal testing device, which I discovered was being used in Germany for measuring skin resistance at acupuncture points. Both were used in the application of what is known as electro-acupuncture.

As I creatively integrated alternative methods of patient evaluation and developed integrative treatment protocols for common issues encountered in my practice, the response of the patients was that they liked the full approach. For them, it was more meaningful and gave them a greater understanding of themselves. They could receive feedback and visually see the changes. Many of the treatments helped to alleviate chronic pain with no drug regimen. I was surprised by the outcome of the treatment results.

A Flourishing Integrative Family Practice

After five years of family practice, I was blessed with an opportunity to buy a large home and property in St. George de Beauce, Québec. This rural town was a center of entrepreneurship in Québec. With the larger house, I had the idea that I could establish my ideal home-based integrative family medical practice. It was a Canadian-style home built on ancestral lands in the 1950s to 1960s, surrounded by an acre of land and trees along the nearby Ruisseau D'Ardoise River. It was a perfect natural, relaxed environment in which to raise my family and further develop my integrative medical practice.

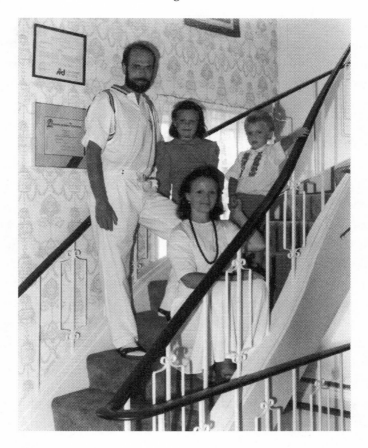

The main floor of the home office included a reception/waiting area and treatment room. In the basement, I set up a homeopathy pharmacy, a Kirlian photo lab, a dark field microscopy lab, a room for electro-acupuncture testing equipment, and a place to grow food hydroponically. It was a place for health and healthy living for my family. The children would often interact with my patients, setting up educational tapes for them to watch and sometimes even offering their own words of advice. My (former) wife Renata, educated in biology and with two years of medical school, was very supportive of my work.

As word spread of my success with integrative medical approaches, my practice flourished and I employed a staff of six. More clients came to see me, after they had been through the traditional medical system of diagnostics and specialists without satisfactory results. Most already had complete lab reports, so I refined my investigative approach to diagnosis and looked at other parameters during the patient exam, in order to form a more complete picture. I evaluated the bioterrain—the biophysical and emotional terrain of the client.

In the early 1990s, I studied dark field microscopy with Dr. Marie Becker of the Enderlein Society in Germany, Dr. Robert Bradford of American Biologics, and Gaston Naessens, a biologist in Sherbrooke, Québec. With dark field microscopy, I was able to do live blood analysis. I looked at a patient's subtle electrical energies with investigative tools, such as Kirlian photography, and used Vega Electro-Dermal testing to take measurements at acupuncture points. With the extra information gained, I was able to develop a more comprehensive integrative protocol for treatment. When someone who was not cured by the regular system comes to you and you help them, they refer others to you. I began to see and treat more and more patients with diseases like chronic fatigue syndrome and cancer.

When someone is diagnosed with cancer, it is a very emotional and dramatic situation. Most people have known someone who has gone through the treatment, and they don't want to go through it themselves. As a family doctor, I did not discourage them from the standard medical treatment. The question wasn't to do or not to do chemotherapy. Some people thought that instead of doing chemotherapy, they could take vitamin C or an all-natural alternative. That was not the case. They needed to be properly informed. Through looking at the whole picture by evaluating their bioterrain, I could discuss with them what resources they had available to handle the tremendous stress that cancer and its treatment would place upon them. We also discussed the potential underlying cause of the cancer. Was it emotional? Nutritional? Due to a pattern of thought and behavior? Were they addicted to anger or something else? This was important, as the removal or shrinking of the cancer itself through medical treatment would not cure the disease itself or address the underlying factors that precipitated it. I tried to give them a full picture of where they were, how they could help themselves through the process, and what tools were available to them. The day that we can put all of the integrative medical resources together for someone going through cancer—that will be a blessing.

Another one of the main problems in medicine I faced as a doctor was the treatment of addictions. Disease is about habits and behaviors that people are addicted to. Whether the addiction is to food or emotions, the path to successful treatment is to change the brain chemistry of someone by teaching them how to create new brain circuits. To help in this, I was already using neurolinguistic programming (NLP) in my treatment approaches. To assist people with smoking cessation, weight loss, and other addictive behaviors, I developed specific integrative treatment protocols that included electro-acupuncture, auriculotherapy, homeopathy, and educational programs on nutrition and behavioral change.

My smoking cessation program included an initial interview in which the treatment was outlined to the client and they were told to immediately stop smoking. A specific point was treated on their ear using auriculotherapy. They were put on a special diet and given homeopathic and other natural products to help detoxify the body and decrease the side effects of withdrawal symptoms. Their habits were discussed and recommendations for behavioral changes were made.

I, like most doctors, didn't have the time to sit and educate my clients on the topics of nutrition and behavior change during a regular visit, so I used a sophisticated S-VHS camera and visual effects to create personalized educational videos for my clients. They could then watch them in a separate viewing room in my house after an appointment or take the videos with them to view at home. This was where my son, Alexi, got his first introduction to filmmaking and A-V equipment, as he would often put the tapes in for the patients.

In the late 1990s, I continued my complementary studies in the field of naturopathy. I received a diploma of naturopathy from the Association des Diplomes en Naturopathie du Québec in 1996 and certification in naturopathy from the American Naturopathic Medical Association in California in 2000.

Over ten years of practice, I had served around 10,000 patients, with little advertising other than a small photo and write-up in the medical directory. My practice had grown largely through referrals, as I had success in implementing complementary treatments for many of the conditions seen by general family practitioners for people of all ages. Some patients even traveled from other parts of the country to see me. By this time, I would say that 90 percent of the prescriptions in my practice were based in natural alternative medicine and only 10 percent were pharmaceuticals.

Over these years of medical practice, I served as vice president of the Holistic Medical Association in Canada, a group of two hundred doctor members. I was also a member of the Association of Naturopaths of Québec and the Professional Union of Homeopaths, and I was later invited to become medical director of the Hypoglycemia Association. I personally became interested in *Candida albicans,* another condition that was unrecognized at the time by the medical establishment, and developed a natural protocol for treatment that included diet and probiotics. Television and radio programs often invited me to speak as a consultant in the areas of hypoglycemia, chronic fatigue, and raw and live food nutrition.

To further my investigation into using dark field microscopy as an evaluation tool, I opened a research lab downtown in the city of Montreal near McGill University. Between my medical practice and lab research, I wanted to investigate the correlation between blood morphology and physiopathologic conditions. Typically, blood morphology is a subjective, qualitative observation. I developed a computer software program for live blood analysis through the compilation of statistics based on specific parameters for viewing. As my work in the lab obtained greater visibility, other doctors began to notice and criticize the complementary alternative approaches I was using in my practice.

I eventually ended my family practice and moved to the United States to participate in a variety of clinical research projects and work as a medical consultant, and I began lecturing in California. From 2002 to 2006, I established and served as president and professor at the Institute of Quantum Biofeedback Naturopathic Medicine (IQBNM) in San Diego, which was accredited by the American Naturopathic Medical Accreditation Board (ANMAB). In 2006, IQBNM became the International Quantum University for Integrative Medicine (IQUIM), known as Quantum University, in Honolulu, Hawaii. This is where I am now focusing my energies in order to share all that I have learned through my own experiences and to promote a new global health-care system of integrative medicine based on the scientific foundation of quantum physics.

Chapter 1
Creating a New Vision for Medicine

Sometimes, when I look back on the screen of my life, I am impressed by the "synchronicity" of events that have guided me until now. Most of the core concepts I refer to today in creative integrative medicine were the very subjects I was attracted to and fascinated by early on, even before medical school.

Psychology was one subject that I explored in depth. When Freud was leaving my favor, I discovered the psychology of the soul with Carl Gustav Jung and immersed myself in the study of everything written by and about him. I pursued research in this area during medical school, and it wasn't surprising that he became the subject of my thesis. Jung's assertion that everything that came to him was from within—an inside-out experience—makes complete sense to me today in light of quantum physics, which describes how objects remain *potentia,* waves of possibility, until they are brought into manifestation through the act of observation. Jung already realized that reality emerges from within. His works on symbolism and archetypes prepared me to better understand the concept of the supramental, later developed by Dr. Amit Goswami, as one body of information in a subtle anatomy.

Synchronicity was another fascinating idea in the Jungian psychology. His collaboration with Wolfgang Pauli connected his work with theories of quantum physics.

Jung and Pauli were convinced that synchronistic events reveal an underlying unity of mind and matter, subjective and objective realities ... Jung and Pauli sought a unifying theory that would allow interpretation of reality as a psycho-physical whole. Pauli thought that probability mathematics expresses physically what is manifested psychologically as archetypes (deep-structured patterns for certain types of universal mental experiences, or patterns of instincts) and synchronistic event (Burns 2011).

When I went to medical school, I was expecting to continue to feed this exploration. Instead, I found myself lost in an environment defined by a materialistic and linear approach toward human beings. I didn't realize it at the time, but I went through a dissociative experience where my unconscious world within didn't fit with what I was discovering outside through my medical studies. It took me years to align my outer reality with the reality within, which I now I express through a new vision for creative integrative medicine.

I had to pursue my inner quest in parallel with my standard studies of medicine by reading and researching what really mattered to me: evolution, the psyche, and consciousness. This is what drew me in my second year of medical school to the practice of yoga and meditation and to the study of consciousness. I had the intuition that these existential questions could not be solved with the mind only. The experience of the fabric of reality had to do with a deeper awareness where all of our being is involved, including the senses, feeling, thinking, and intuition. At that time, the subject of yoga was not very popular and meditation was even less so. These practices, that many clinicians suggest to their patients for stress release today, were described back then as being in conflict with the Christian faith and weren't very popular.

It took me years to integrate these different traditions. It was very enlightening later on when I read *The Tao of Physics* by Capra (1975). He correlated the way mystics and longtime contemplatives and meditators were describing reality with how quantum physics also perceived it. This introduces us to a completely different interpretation of our perception of reality.

Before I could envision a clear path for an integrative medicine practice, I had to experience altered states of consciousness through different meditation practices, I also traveled all over the world to discover that I was not the only one on this journey, which brought me to my sabbatical year in Switzerland, where other medical doctors from different continents interested in the studies of meditation, relaxation, consciousness, and quantum physics came together. Very few people know that Maharishi Mahesh Yogi, founder of transcendental meditation, was also a physicist and pioneer in his work, correlating quantum physics and consciousness. Through this very special yearlong experience, I was exposed to his vision and research. It was just before Dr. Deepak Chopra joined him. After that year, I didn't know exactly how this fundamental experience of altered states of awareness and consciousness studies would be implemented in my practice. Holistic medicine wasn't really known in Canada until a few years later.

As mentioned earlier, many years passed during which my integrative medical practice took on many forms. But there was still a missing link to bridge the gap and bring all of this information together. One day in 2004, I, like many other practitioners in this emerging field of quantum medicine, was surprised by the movie *What the Bleep Do We Know?!* (Arntz 2004). This was my first introduction to Dr. Amit Goswami and all of the other featured scientists who have since become so popular. I couldn't take my mind off one of Goswami's statements in the film. He said, "Consciousness is the ground of everything." Gerber, with his book *Vibrational Medicine* (1988), was already pointing in this direction—to the emerging points of view of quantum physics. But when all of these renowned quantum physicists began connecting this information to the recent research in neurobiology, I think everybody interested in this subject had a moment.

At the time, I made many attempts to have one of these eminent scientists do some work in conjunction with the university I had established, but I was unsuccessful. Then I just let it go. A few years later, while surfing on the Web, I discovered the book *The Quantum Doctor* (Goswami 2004) and ordered it immediately. I didn't realize that the author, Dr. Amit Goswami, was the *same* scientist in the *Bleep* movie that had captured my mind with his line "Consciousness is the ground of everything." His book *The Quantum Doctor* signified for me the beginning of an enlightening journey during which I went through several epiphanies. I rediscovered through reading this book (and all of his other books) the main subjects that had been at the center of my quest for so many years.

I finally contacted him, and from there, we began developing what is today the foundation for the curriculum of creative integrative medicine that we teach at Quantum University. We believe that in a few years, it will be adopted as the premise for many medical university curriculums.

Dr. Goswami, through his foundational work, has in my perspective laid out the scientific ground for modern medicine and pushed the boundaries of previous pioneers of quantum medicine, such as Dr. Deepak Chopra. The alternative modalities that have belonged to the domains of health spas, relaxation, or personal growth can now be integrated within the medical arena because of his insights into quantum physics and its relation to the art of healing.

Through my own process of spiritual awakening, triggered by the dramatic event of my brother's death, I see today that the realization of my founding of Quantum University is the manifestation of my inner world vision into an outer reality. I had been seeking to express a new, improved foundation for medicine wherein the infinite possibilities of healing can be expressed to allow any individual facing disease and suffering to hope for a full potential of health.

Asking the Question: How Do We Heal?

I will never forget a particular consultation early on in my rural medical practice. One day, a lady with immense stature and confidence walked into my office. She was the wife of a farmer and her language was straightforward and unequivocal. She confidently strode in and sat solidly down in the consultation chair, looked directly into my eyes, and said, "Doctor, you are not the one who heals here. The Lord is the one." Honestly, I did not know what to do with this.

A few years later on a Saturday afternoon—one of those days where you try to catch up with your weekend gardening—a patient called me out of the blue. She belonged to a prayer group and was organizing a special prayer meeting for a friend of hers, Paul Remy, who was in a very critical state in the intensive care unit at the hospital. I didn't know Paul Remy, but he was very popular and beloved in the area. He was a man of great esteem who had many children and grandchildren, who had labored on his farm all of his life, and who had the reputation of an unshakable faith. I was not completely familiar with this type of prayer experience, but I was curious and open to any kind of spiritual experience that could help to deepen my understanding. I had to go to that neighborhood anyway, to buy some necessities at the hardware store, so I thought, *Why not pass by and see what's going on?*

The meeting was happening in a back room of a church. It was filthy, packed with people, and heating up with prayers. This type of prayer group, known as a charismatic prayer group, was starting to gain popularity in Québec. I believe it was an expression, within a Catholic environment, of what is very popular in some American churches. It left an impression on me, since it was the first time I had been exposed to so much fervor.

During the process, something amazing began to happen. I started to feel some heat rise within me as a member of the group spoke about the need for someone to be chosen to go to the hospital to pray for Paul Remy. I was very embarrassed by this situation as the heat within continued to amplify and some unusual feelings crept in. I just tried to hide so that nobody could recognize that I was going through some type of noticeable experience. But it reached a point where this was not possible anymore, and it appeared obvious that I was the one who must go to visit Paul Remy.

I didn't know him at all, and I had to go to the hospital where everybody knew me. This was surely not what I had planned for the day. I wanted to rush out of there and resist their request. As if there were not already enough unusual circumstances for the day, when I got into my car, a cold, autumn wind brought to my feet a palm tree branch. There were many subsequent occasions when I continued to ask myself where this palm tree branch had come from, as they did not grow here in Québec. But the synchronicity of this event gave me the extra courage I needed to go to the hospital.

When I got there, I was informed that Paul Remy was in intensive care. His diagnosis listed a heart attack, pulmonary embolism, and cardiac failure. With this combination of medical problems, the statistical odds of someone surviving are almost zero. I walked into his room where he was half-conscious and proceeded quickly to carry out my mission.

In the days following, Paul Remy recuperated from his impossible situation and later became a great friend. Of course, I don't take any credit for this healing, but today I realize that this event was one of spontaneous healing, an event that can only be explained through the principles of quantum physics, as you will discover later on in this book.

Further on in my medical career, I was invited to a convention in Switzerland where doctors from all over the world came together to explore one main question: who heals? There were as many answers to that question as there were participants. Years later, as I watched a sci-fi movie called *K-PAX*, I was struck by a passage spoken by the main character. "For your information, every being has the capacity to cure themselves" (Softley 2001).

So who does the healing? What the lady who had walked into my office expressed to me years ago, and what this charismatic prayer group made me experience so dramatically is what many of our ancestors have known for generations—that there is another unseen element involved in healing that goes beyond a doctor's prescription. Today, quantum physicists, such as Dr. Goswami, describe this unseen element as consciousness. Dr. Goswami purports that consciousness is "the ground of all being," the source from which healing comes (1997).

Many studies have shown that prayer can heal at a distance, and nonlocality is one of the principles of quantum physics that supports an explanation of this phenomenon. Complementary modalities of healing can also be explained through quantum physics, but to understand this will require a shift in the experience of reality.

Even at that time, when I was searching and curious about different modalities of healing, I was still imprinted by a linear way of thinking that these experiences couldn't necessarily fit into. It's one thing to read and learn about quantum physics and consciousness; it is quite another to experience a new perspective from within. I believe that over the last thirty years, many of us have been, in some way, apprentices in the exploration of new approaches to healing—guided most of the time by intuition. All of the pieces of the puzzle began to come together for me when a new scientific understanding of the fabric of reality was put in place by a generation of quantum physicists that had the courage to translate this knowledge into the world of medicine. Dr. Amit Goswami is certainly of them. As I will explain below, it literally turns our whole perspective of the world upside down.

An Evolving Scientific View of Reality

One of the major sources of resistance I met on my medical journey, when integrating diverse modalities of healing, was the notion that these modalities were not based on science and for that reason were not taught in Western medical schools. When I started to look more closely at these arguments, I realized, like others, that what we define as science is very relative. I also became aware that our choices of scientific perspective as a society have most often been associated with a conflict of interest. I was shocked to realize how our way of thinking is complicated by the world's sociopolitical interests. The pretention of being objective and scientific has nothing to do with being objective and scientific. In fact, how scientists, philosophers, and theologians have experienced and described reality has evolved over time and will be forever changing.

This concept of how we experience reality was already one of the existential questions I reflected on as a teenager. As I said earlier, the death of my brother had evoked in me this quest to understand the how and the why of things. I was born and raised with a very traditional Catholic background. My academic success in school allowed me to pursue my secondary school studies at a Catholic seminary where I was exposed to the study of Latin, Greek, existential, and Christian philosophies, and the sciences.

Early on, I became interested in French philosophical literature. Blaise Pascal (1623–1662), a scientist and philosopher who wrote, "The heart has its reason which reason does not know" (Pascal 1669), was among my favorites. He was already discussing the underlying dichotomy of experience between the senses and the mind. Sometimes, I would retreat for days into nature, bringing with me lectures on philosophy, literature, psychology, spirituality, and science. I became intrigued by how, throughout history, philosophers, scientists, and theologians have dealt with how to integrate spirituality and science together and have attempted to solve the issue of dichotomy between mind and body.

Four hundred years ago, Galileo's challenge of Copernicanism was controversial within his lifetime. Galileo was eventually forced to recant his heliocentrism and spent the last years of his life under house arrest on orders of the Roman Inquisition. Today, everybody smiles about that story, but at that time it was taken very seriously. Changing the perspective of how we looked at the world had enormous consequences, not only religiously but also sociopolitically.

Now history is repeating itself; another landmark shift in human perspective of the reality of the universe is occurring. Over time, our understanding of the mechanics of the universe has guided us to develop the societal structures we are now experiencing in these modern times. When quantum physics came along in the last century, we could not predict all of the ripple effects that this new awareness of the fabric of reality would create. Unfortunately, one of the first applications of it was for nuclear energy used for destructive purposes. Since then, quantum physics has continued to slowly permeate all stratums of society.

Applying a Quantum Perspective to Evolution and Biology

A major query that drew me toward science and biology was the question of evolution. As many others tried to inject the idea of purposefulness into creation, Darwin's opinion no longer satisfied my mind. Pierre Teilhard de Chardin (1881–1955), a French philosopher, Jesuit priest, paleontologist, and geologist, was one who certainly began to lay out an integrative vision for a new biology. His concepts of *biosphere, noosphere,* and *Christosphere* (revised in the context of quantum physics by Goswami in his book *God Is Not Dead* (2008), could be considered today prophetic. The church initially opposed his views but has since gradually begun to look at them more favorably.

> Teilhard's position was opposed by his Church superiors and some of his work was denied publication during his lifetime by the Roman Holy Office. The 1950 encyclical *Humani Generis* condemned several of Teilhard's opinions, while leaving other questions open. However, some of Teilhard's views became influential in the

reforms of the Second Vatican Council. More recently, Pope John Paul II indicated a positive attitude towards some of Teilhard's ideas. In 2009, Pope Benedict XVI mentioned Teilhard's idea of the universe as a "living host (*Wikipedia*)."

Purposefulness in evolution is at the core of what we today call a new biology—one based on the primacy of consciousness and quantum physics, as introduced by Dr. Goswami. The science of life, frozen in the old view of Darwinism (where evolution is driven by the survival of the fittest), has resulted in the generation of a fatalistic model of medicine where there is no room for regeneration, spontaneous healing, or even higher quality of life. How we understand evolution has a lot to do with how we perceive disease, which most of the time (especially for chronic diseases) is a situation for which there is no solution. A given fatalistic diagnosis will not be defined in terms of healing but rather in terms of how much time someone has left to live or what treatments can alleviate the symptoms. With this approach, there is no cure for the cause or possibility of stepping outside the box that the patient has been put in for the rest of their life.

Through further extracurricular studies, it became very clear to me that universities and medical schools have an urgent need to update their curriculum from such a limiting model of evolution to a new biology that can sustain new modalities and perspectives on healing and bring consciousness into biology. The old biology depicting the human being as a machine in a mechanical world of inanimate objects, with symptomatic approaches to healing, must be replaced by a positive science of life. This gives us a basis for integrative medicine that can treat disease by healing emotional blocks and self-limiting mental constructs, including quantum leaps of intuition and theories of creative evolution.

A new view of biology can lead to the creation of a scientific environment within which we acknowledge the possibility for an intelligent design, spontaneous healing, creativity, subjectivity, and heterogeneity. Consciousness can be seen as the information source guiding the growth of our bodies, a blueprint of the world for all time. It is the force which must be tapped into in order to heal. In a new biology, the goal will not be survival of the fittest but rather a striving toward more sophisticated representations, more complex forms of life correlated with new morphogenetic fields, and new brain circuits. (We will be discussing this topic in more detail in a later chapter.)

Fundamentally, this idea of a new biology, when combined with the application of other principles of quantum physics to medicine, will turn the existing scientific world's perception of causation and creation upside down.

In quantum physics, there are no manifest material objects independent of subjects: the observers. In other words, matter (as defined in terms of elementary particles of atoms, molecules, and cells) is explained by the fundamental premise that everything can be described in terms of possibilities. Dr. Goswami has expressed this concept as "consciousness as the ground of all being." In his book *The Quantum Doctor*, he describes in detail this shift from an upward causation model (matter first) through to a downward causation model (consciousness first). When you start to apply this new paradigm shift to medicine, you soon have vertigo.

> Quantum physics has shifted our perspective of reality from a linear materialistic model to a multidimensional model of consciousness. This turns the existing scientific world's perception of causation and creation upside down, opening the door to new possibilities in how we perceive factors governing biology, evolution, psychology, and medicine (Goswami 2004).

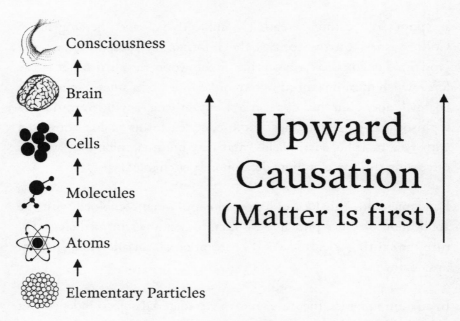

Figure 1.1: Upward Causation (Quantum Doctor Course)

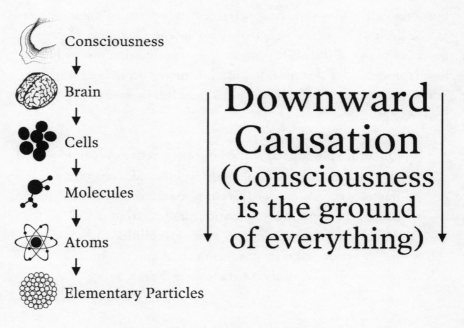

Figure 1.2: Downward Causation (Quantum Doctor Course)

At a Crossroads: Creating a New Model for Healing

Conventional medicine, to date, has been definitively based on the linear and materialistic point of view of the upward causation model. This has resulted in a model of healing where the only legitimate therapies are pharmaceuticals, surgery, and other physical therapies. Therefore, anything that could be related to as subtle energy (prana, ch'i, vital force) could not be scientifically justified as a valid approach to healing within this model. This is as simple as it gets. Even today, no matter how many studies are published on the benefits of complementary medical approaches, they will continue to be disregarded because their fundamental basis is not a materialistic one.

Today, everybody is aware of the worldwide energy crisis. There is a dramatic awakening to the fact that we can't continue to rely on oil as a sole source of energy generation. Not only is this dependence on oil related to pollution, but it also has political, economic, and social consequences. Countries may have different strategies, but everybody is now looking at other sources of energy, such as solar and wind.

In the domain of medicine, we are facing a similar crossroads. We are using an outdated model of science that can only support conventional Western modalities of healing, the costs of which are exorbitant and unsustainable. Conventional medicine continues to face challenges in the understanding and effective treatment of chronic disease. We can't deny the progress of a symptomatic approach, but studies have shown that chronic disease consumes the majority of the health-care budget. Seventy-six percent of Medicare spending is on patients with one of five or more chronic diseases (Swartz 2010).

By shifting our perspective to a downward causation model, we will create a new therapeutic reality where alternative medical treatments can be understood and integrated with allopathic medicine. It is important to realize how critical this discussion is. Modern medicine will never welcome alternative, complementary, or integrative treatments without a model of understanding that provides a common scientific foundation for all forms of medicine.

Challenges in Implementing Integrative Medicine

As a doctor, I was successful in integrating some complementary approaches into my medical practice that satisfied the needs of many patients, including those who were unable to be helped by the traditional system. However, in doing so, I faced controversy from those who argued that alternative methods do not belong in the practice of a medical doctor on the basis that they are not scientific and are not taught in medical school. Peer pressure within the medical community continues to discourage the use of alternative methods. Why should people facing pain and suffering not have alternative sources of healing? People have already been searching outside the system and paying out of their own pockets for alternative treatments.

While some hospitals and clinics are now putting out banners for integrative medicine and offering acupuncture, massage, nutrition, and other treatments, they are doing so without being taught about them in medical school as part of an integrative model for medicine. Acupuncture, for example, has been accepted on the basis of its use in pain management and stimulation of endorphins, but without regard for the basic concepts of the five elements and ch'i in Chinese medicine. While naturopathic doctors are trained in natural medicine, homeopathy, nutrition, and other natural remedies, they typically use an allopathic and Western philosophy-based approach.

In order to be successful in implementing integrative medicine, it will be necessary to address the following key issues.

- Address the current health-care crisis and unsustainable rising health-care costs by providing alternative protocols, particularly for people who cannot afford surgery or pharmaceuticals.

- Establish the credibility of alternative therapies within the scientific community and gain recognition by medical boards for their use. This can be done through the creation of a new paradigm of integrative medicine based on the science of quantum physics, to be taught at medical schools.

- Recognize an expanded view of the anatomy of a human body, which includes the mind-body connection and subtle energy fields.

- Develop new approaches to client evaluation and diagnosis using additional tools of investigation in order to provide a holistic view of the person.

- Redefine a model for modern medicine based on the principles of quantum physics that creates a new environment for healing focused not on disease but on how to optimize the full potential of the human being.

Integrative medicine is not just a new cosmetic name for complementary alternative medicine; that term should also imply the premise of inclusion of conventional medicine. The responsibility in the future for medical universities will be to include in their curriculum the essential knowledge of a more complex understanding of the fabric of the reality of the human being, one based on an understanding of the science of quantum physics and a philosophy of potential versus fatality.

Finding a Solution to Today's Health-Care Crisis

As a new doctor in the 1970s in Canada, I was excited about the promise of social medicine. Now, years later, I have a different perspective and have seen how a heavy bureaucracy has taken over the management of health care. Administrators with no medical knowledge have made decisions based on cost reduction that have greatly impacted patient care. Patients now wait a long time to receive proper care. A doctor's freedom of practice has also been compromised. There is no longer one doctor responsible for a patient; the personal connection has been lost. Nobody is "in charge" of the patient or has a complete vision, a holistic picture of what is going on. There is no sense of total responsibility anymore. Most often, the general practitioner relies on what the specialist perceives. But how can we rely on that when the specialists are only looking at a small piece of the picture? Today's philosophy of health care is fractured.

The diagnostic approach used in conventional Western medicine puts the patient in a mode where there is no possibility of overcoming their doctor's stated outcome, such as happened to my own brother. It is a fear-based, fatalistic view, which places the patient in a helpless position.

When I moved to America, I discovered there were also many flaws in the health-care system here. Even if reform is necessary, there is unfortunately no questioning of how medicine is practiced or how to change the fundamental approach to healing to make it more affordable and available to everybody.

In my own journey, when I learned how a new scientific foundation for medicine based on the principles of quantum physics could create a new environment for healing, I began to look at everything from a different point of view—a point of view that everything is possible, a perspective from which full potential could redefine modern medicine.

The old family doctor, such as the one we had for my brother, knew the whole family and took responsibility for my brother's care when others wouldn't. This made a significant impression in my life and on my role as a doctor. It is my hope that creative integrative medicine will bring back the old traditional role of family doctor, that the creative integrative doctor will be one who looks at the whole person, takes total responsibility for their care, and approaches the situation from the viewpoint of potential instead of one of fatalistic limitations.

Chapter 2
Quantum Creativity: Exploring the Science behind Spontaneous Healing

Commonalities among Spontaneous Healing Experiences

The idea of spontaneous healing related to consciousness, as brought forth by Dr. Deepak Chopra with his best-selling 1990s book *Quantum Healing* (1989), revolutionized the world of quantum medicine. He noted, unexpectedly, that patients who physicians had discarded or predicted a fatal outcome for would heal after experiencing a new awareness about their situation. A vocabulary emerged to describe the workings of these "magical" healings as a "quantum leap of awareness." This was not a new phenomenon, nor was it one that medicine may have tagged as wrongly diagnosed, previously eliminated, or resulting from an error in filling out the patient's information. These sporadic events had already been common knowledge throughout the history of humanity. In another time, we called them miraculous healings and left the scientific community out of it when they didn't have the capacity to understand what was really going on.

But today, what if I were to tell you that the science for quantum healing is available and that this knowledge makes perfect sense according to the views of modern quantum physics? Not only that, but we can teach you a step-by-step approach to make these events more likely to occur. Who would not be interested in this knowledge? If you are involved in the study of natural or alternative medicine, or you are a medical doctor or other health-care professional facing the limits of conventional cures on a daily basis, would you not be curious about this? Why should this not be taught at medical schools—the science of healing—as part of a curriculum for natural and integrative medicine, or at least as a perspective on the healing of disease that provides an alternative to a fatalistic prognosis?

Since Dr. Chopra's book *Quantum Healing*, many patients, doctors, and writers have added their testimonies to this phenomenon. Certainly, Dr. Goswami, in his book *The Quantum Doctor*, has contributed a major piece of the scientific foundation for and understanding of quantum healing, with the added concept of quantum creativity.

It was a priority for me to embed this critical information and more into a comprehensive curriculum, pushing the frontier of a new model of health-care education. This understanding of the science of spontaneous healing is being taught in order to bring a new breadth of healing and quantum insight into the health-care field to give health-care professionals the opportunity to explore new creative approaches and expand our understanding of what leads to a permanent cure for disease.

I have thought that any phenomena of spontaneous healing or stories of patients healed spontaneously should be considered as a testimony in favor of quantum medicine. I understood that even if these stories didn't have the validity of scientific research, they could inspire many health-care practitioners and patients who had been given a fatalistic diagnosis. As a result, my son, Alexi, and I decided to spread the good news by creating a new online channel called Quantum World TV. We were motivated both by this purpose and by being able to invite to our program renowned doctors or clinicians who could contribute to quantum medicine. You can see many of these recorded events online at http://iquim.org/quantum-world-tv/.

One of these programs tells the incredible story of Gulie and again shows how the universe's play can involve many actors, leaving everyone with the recognition that what is happening is beyond the ego. In the previous conventional model of healing, the doctor is invested with a tremendous amount of power, often leaving the patient powerless. In quantum medicine, as the health-care practitioner matures, he or she realizes that here the mechanics really are quite different. Behind the scenes, The Watcher (what Gulie named her healing source) is guiding her every step of the way.

Gulie's Story

I first called Gulie out of the blue after an online homotoxicology class. This is something I never do because of limited time availability, but in her case, I felt I couldn't properly answer her question at the end of the class for confidentiality reasons. This call led me to refer Gulie to a friend, a homeopathic pharmacist in Québec, after suggesting that her hair analysis revealed a serious arsenic toxicity. She was in a state of shock, realizing that she had been poisoned. She took care of the arsenic poisoning through detoxification but later went on to develop breast cancer.

Again, for no special reason other than to inquire about her health, I called her and she sadly informed me of her new situation. I realized that she was trying to face this new challenge all by herself. We will speak later in this chapter about the optimal conditions for spontaneous healing, but one important factor is to create a momentum that will allow for a leap of awareness about the conflicted emotions related to cancer or disease. In her case, it was anger. The challenge is not just to identify the conflict but also to discover how to experience a deep release of the emotion.

Through experience, I knew that the probability for this to occur would be much higher if the client was in a therapeutic relationship. I had witnessed many clients who had come for evaluation erroneously thinking that they had worked out the conflict associated with their disease but who were in reality still at the surface of it. This can eventually carry one to a critical state of health. This is not a situation to be dealt with lightly and needs to be taken care of with a lot of professionalism and competency, which is why it is so imperative that complementary medicine and conventional medicine work together under the same roof, under the banner of integrative medicine.

So I referred her to one of my dear students, Dr. Wendy Rudell, who knew how to integrate the concepts of quantum medicine with live foods nutritional counseling. Gulie's health problems required a multifaceted approach combining nutrition, detoxification, and resolution of the associated conflict. I invite you to hear and see the happy ending of her story online at http://iquim.org/quantum-world-tv/wendy-rudell/june-19-2010/.

Before we go more deeply into the mechanics of quantum healing, let me tell you another extraordinary story. In some way, all of the stories with my patients/clients through time have been love stories. I can remember the special circumstances under which I met each of them for the first time. Dea is another one of them.

Dea's Story

This touching story will reveal the complexity of emotional conflicts that can be related to breast cancers, which often occur in more than one generation in a family. These conflicts look like a crystal with multiple facets, and when we think that the conflict has been solved, it may reappear from another angle. This brings us to one of the major challenges encountered in spontaneous healing: how to stabilize the healing event, as it appears in the sparkle of an ah-ha moment, in the neurophysiology and physicality of an individual. This is what Dr. Goswami calls "creating new brain circuits," a concept that is supported by the emerging science of neuroplasticity.

Dea was the wife of a pastor of a small Christian community in Oregon. Diagnosed with breast cancer, she decided to have a local removal of the tumor without extensive surgery and complemented the surgery with a natural approach based on supplements and nutrition. To be more aggressive at the beginning with her natural therapies, she went for an intensive detox and orthomolecular treatment at a medical health clinic in Mexico.

The first time we met was at this medical health clinic in Mexico. She was in her late fifties. She was doing very well at this time, especially after the extensive detoxification and hyper-vitamin therapy that she received at this clinic. Throughout her treatment, Dea was continuously supervised by her medical doctor and had many lab tests or radiology exams as tumor markers, as required by her condition. I served as her educator and coach, not her medical doctor. I was the one who guided her along the way on her healing path while she continued to be under her own doctor's medical supervision.

Surprisingly, her daughter, who was in her late thirties, had also been diagnosed with the same type of cancer. Choosing not to share the same fate as her mother, she decided to be treated entirely with conventional medicine.

The conflict associated with Dea's breast cancer was what we call a nest conflict, or in the terminology of Hamer medicine, "a family conflict." Her most recent conflicting situation had happened within the community with another community member. She thought of this other member as her own daughter and was very affected by the event, having a sense of devaluation associated with it. Strangely, her biological daughter was going through a similar conflict, but within a different scenario. The daughter was not open to any introspection and was cultivating an attitude of victim regarding her past trauma. Dea, even though she was older, had a remarkable ability for introspection and was very open to working with techniques such as quantum biofeedback, visualization, and neurolinguistics.

For many years, while still under supervision for tumor markers for the cancer, Dea's recovery appeared to be well under control. Her cancer was considered to have been in remission for almost five years. At the same time, her daughter continued to deteriorate. As I became more involved with the development of the university and had less time availability, Dea began seeing a naturopathic doctor who was more nutritionally oriented, and I lost contact with her for another year or two. One day, I called her to inquire how things were going. Unfortunately, this time another emotional trauma with her own mother had triggered, from another angle, her sense of devaluation, and the cancer had recurred. An impressive mass was visible in her right armpit. (Pictures are available in the new quantum medicine course at Quantum University.)

This type of event is very important and meaningful in the management of cancer patients. It doesn't matter if the approach is a natural or strictly medical one; all patients should be investigating the emotional component that could be associated with the cancer or other disease. One of the major problems inherent in the follow-up of cancer patients is the fear that the cancer can recur. Even after radiotherapy and chemotherapy, most cancer patients will be followed with the tragic expectation of "Why could this cancer not come back again, since the real underlying cause of the problem has not been taken care of by a symptomatic approach?"

I am not saying that we have found the cause of cancers in complementary medicine, but there are certainly risk factors that appear more and more evident. The emotional component is one of them, and the toxicity of the bioterrain is another one. The language of conventional medicine most often discourages patients from saying that these components have anything to do with cancer. This view is similar to that of heavily smoking surgeons and pneumologists treating lung cancer who, when I was doing my medical residency, were saying that tobacco had not been proven to cause cancer.

Another important factor here is the risk of assuming that the business of solving conflicts takes care of everything. This could easily be another trap—to think that the patient can, through some kind of mind fantasy, completely ignore the supervision of competent medical doctors. Creative integrative medicine should ultimately bring the best of both approaches together.

I also want to insist that in Dea's case, even though she had done a lot of work to manage her original conflict, in her situation that would not have meant *game over*. A conflict can appear in a different scenario and carry with it the same theme—in her case, a sense of devaluation. This is why the client should, in these situations, be equipped with different techniques, such as neurolinguistic programming (NLP) or emotional freedom technique (EFT). These techniques use visualizations or meditations to help prevent a situation from retriggering past memories. I believe that the next chapter of medicine will be written by the science of neuroplasticity and the ability to create new neurologic pathways associated with new behaviors in regard to our past trauma(s).

But let us come back to our story that was taking a much more dramatic turn. The recurrence of the cancer alarmed Dea, and in observing this voluminous mass, she decided to see her doctor who began radiotherapy again to at least shrink the mass. I invited her to visit me in San Diego between her treatments. She went through some sessions of quantum biofeedback and some visualizations to help release the stress associated with this frightening situation. She went back home, and there something unexpected happened: the mass literally fell off her armpit like a bunch of grapes. I had heard similar stories of spontaneous healing in the past that I just couldn't believe. This time, it happened with the evidence of pictures that I couldn't deny. When she visited the hospital, the nurses would identify her as "the one that happened to." However, the medical doctor who was doing the follow-up took all the credit and touted it as another victory for radiotherapy, even though the most common side effects of that are swelling; small red marks; and darker, firmer, or shrinking breast tissue rather than what actually occurred.

When I saw her again, this time in Hawaii, we recorded her on video with tears in her eyes as she expressed her gratitude. Yet she was torn because her daughter had just died from the same type of breast cancer.

At the time of this video, Dea had survived her cancer for almost ten years more than was expected in her case. This is the ending for now of a chapter of her life that I will have to pursue in another book. You can find the detailed presentation of her case online in the new quantum medicine class at Quantum University.

Bruce Feiler's Healing Journey

It's important to recognize that spontaneous healing is not the property of a specific type of medicine—either natural or conventional. These events can happen in many different contexts. One day while I was listening to CNN, I saw the amazing story of a father of two daughters, Bruce Feiler, who had been diagnosed with an osteosarcoma of his left femur (Gupta 2010).

Today, cancer free, he revealed his enlightening journey that took him through what we call in the world of quantum medicine ah-ha moments, which revealed to him a completely new awareness about what life is. He belongs to a very elite group of only two known survivors of the same medical condition in the entire world. During the time of his awakening, while he created what he calls "the Council of Dads" to provide for his daughters the presence they would miss if he died, he was also being treated with extensive conventional medical care that was certainly essential to his healing.

Listening to this incredible story, I couldn't help but see behind the curtain a bigger play, where an individual was expanding his awareness to a greater reality. In his testimony, Bruce said something like "While becoming less human through all of the aggressive therapies, I was at the same time becoming more human than ever." What he shares in his book *The Council of Dads* (2010), which I highly recommend, are his many insights which happened along this difficult path; they changed both him and his family and I am sure were part of his own healing. You can find more details about his story online at http://councilofdads. ning.com/ or in his book *The Council of Dads*.

Working within a Greater Reality

I have illustrated through these stories some of the challenges we meet in spontaneous healing. These phenomena are no longer isolated events. You will find many of them online or in the literature of quantum medicine. This doesn't mean that they are completely understood or can be reproduced automatically. It's not as simple as taking a pill. I used to say in conferences, "Everybody wants to go to heaven, but no one likes to die." This means that this sort of experience usually requires of the client a letting go of what they see as a survival element within the limited reality they are caught in.

To help understand this, I will use the example of an alcoholic. Everybody agrees with the negative aspects of this addiction. The path that someone has to go through to quit the alcohol addiction is not always an easy one. Alcoholics Anonymous has figured out a twelve-step path, where the individual first must surrender to a *greater power* than himself and associate with forgiveness for himself and others; all of this laborious processing will be successful only if the new choice of sobriety is reinforced on a daily basis by prayer and frequent group meetings.

Quantum healing seems new for many, but essentially what we are speaking about is close to the same thing. Surrendering to a reality greater than I is certainly a common denominator. The difference is that, most of the time, conflicts are related to more subtle addictive emotions, and these emotions have a different tone or angle. In the example of Dea, the general theme was devaluation of self. Nobody will ever doubt that devaluing oneself can be as destructive an addiction as alcohol. Everybody knows her as having a tender heart, always considering others before herself. In other words, the work of the creative integrative doctor will be to explore, with the help of a coach or psychotherapist and with the same scrutiny with which we assess the tumor, the nature of the conflicts or emotions involved in any type of disease with a psychosomatic component—cancer being at the top of the list.

The Importance of Intention in Healing

In quantum medicine, the intention of the healer is crucial. The whole process must be based on a proper intention. More precisely, in regard to the entanglement between the observer and the subject (the client), the outcome of healing can be influenced by the belief system and the intention of the doctor. Many individuals diagnosed with a fatal disease have been able to counteract the negativity and the limited view of conventional medicine, but this requires a lot of character and determination and is not an optimal situation. Most of the time, the patient can only go as far as the perspective imposed by the mainstream.

Along my own journey as a medical doctor, I have experienced how my view has progressively evolved toward the infinite possibilities for healing. Caught at the beginning by the deterministic aspect of a diagnosis, my perception has continued to expand toward a multidimensional reality not revealed by linear materialism, one where I can tap into many layers of information (as described earlier) in order to trigger the process of restoration. This is not just a virtual concept. During my practice, I witnessed many case stories of patients who, if not totally cured, were improved by these complementary approaches. I came to realize that no matter who walked into my office, I had the firm conviction that anything was possible. The result could be expected or not, but in the end, there was healing.

Quantum healing, when it is really understood, makes the doctor or practitioner realize that they are not at the center of this event (this probably reminds you of Copernicus) but that the client or patient, grounded in the fundamental reality of consciousness healing, is. I am grateful to my clients and patients who have revealed to me the infinite possibilities of healing—from seemingly small to fatal conditions. Surprisingly, my colleagues didn't share the same excitement. I learned, at my own expense, that healing in conventional medicine is not always the main target. Or if it is, it must follow a set of rules that can't accept anything outside of the medical protocol.

One of my dear teachers in homeopathy, more precisely in homotoxicology, would often say in defense of homeopathy, "The one who heals is the one who is right." I will admit that it was obviously not the most scientific statement, but still, it reflects some common sense. After I had been practicing homeopathy for a few years as part of my integrative medical practice, a man came to consult with me for a difficult problem. A diagnosed diabetic for many years, he had developed a very bad lesion on one of his feet. This lesion was not healing even though he was receiving all of the standard medical attention he could, with intensive care of the infected area. After the orthopedic surgeon advised him that the next step would be amputation, he followed the advice of his friends and came to visit me.

I listened attentively to his story and suggested some typical homeopathy suitable for his condition. I didn't expect much and didn't want to create impossible expectations in his mind. However, I asked him to be very discrete no matter what the results were, since I knew the orthopedic surgeon and didn't want to be the object of criticism. Plus I knew that if the patient improved, that still would not be enough to convince the surgeon of the benefits of homeopathy.

A few weeks later, the client came back for a consult and, exceeding all my expectations, his foot was no longer at risk for an amputation. In his enthusiasm from the result, he attempted to convert the orthopedic surgeon to homeopathy. But as expected, the specialist, overwhelmed by his scientific superiority, just had a big laugh. Why would he not at least be curious and investigate what could have made the difference? Because what mattered to him was to follow the standard recognized and accepted model of conventional healing. Sadly, a medical doctor will often expose himself to reprimand by his peers and lawsuits if he ventures outside of the mainstream.

Intention is central to quantum healing and, as we have just seen, we may assume that the common intention of any system of healing is to heal. Intention, to be working at its best, cannot be diluted by any other agenda except an act of compassion with detachment. In an interview with Dr. Goswami, in the context of the quantum doctor course, I asked him many questions regarding this important subject. If the medical care system as we know it is not the most supportive environment, the field of energetic medicine can sometimes be out of alignment with the most favorable strategy. In this interview with Dr. Goswami, some interesting points came out. For example, the more the intention is individualized and personally related to, the more it seems to provide a better result. Some energetic healers, excited by the nonlocality of an energetic device, may fill their computer software with a list of clients with the goal of implementing many therapies at once for many people. This is certainly not the best understanding of intention either. No matter how powerful a computer is, none at this point have the capacity to provide the meaning for what is processed. Only the mind has the capacity to do that, according to Dr. Goswami. In other words, the healer, through consciousness, certainly is a big part of this equation. In the model of quantum medicine, we are not going in the direction of an automatic and impersonal medicine; we are doing the opposite. In some ways, the old family doctor was probably closer to this model than the modern one who has to function in a more legalistic, bureaucratic, and standardized environment, one that doesn't allow for creativity.

How Incorporating Quantum Creativity Can Contribute to the Healing Process

Quantum medicine continues to bring more details to the mechanics of healing as revealed by quantum physics. Dr. Goswami has once again pushed the boundaries of this comprehension by adding the core concept of quantum creativity. It is described as four stages: preparation, incubation, sudden insight, and manifestation.

I refer the reader again, for more details, to the book *The Quantum Doctor*, whose content has been further refined in the development of classes that are now part of the curriculum at Quantum University.

One of the major realizations I have had related to this matter of creativity is that we are dealing with a client/patient that isn't a disease per se but someone who is the subject within which an imbalance has been manifested and within whom this manifestation can be reversed. The technology of quantum healing resides in the understanding that a client himself or herself is being entangled with another awareness: the practitioner/doctor who will play an important role in guiding this process.

Ideally, the doctor/practitioner will provide the best environment or the optimal conditions for these creative events to occur in. When you look closely at these conditions, however, you see that the conventional model of medicine most often doesn't provide them. Sometimes, the field of natural medicine, by reproducing the same model of thinking as conventional medicine, also makes *un faux pas* when setting up a new model for healing.

To make something new happen (healing), something different has to be done. Dr. Chopra, in his book *Quantum Healing*, describes the quantum leap as "a new awareness about the reality in which the client could be caught and has created this deadly condition" (Chopra 1989). In the movie *What the Bleep Do We Know?!* this phenomenon is well illustrated, adding in the understanding of emotional chemistry that is associated with it. Many have also described a correlation of conflicts that could be associated with different diseases. Louise Hay is certainly a pioneer in this regard. More recently, and not without controversy.

Preparation

Before we even touch on the substance of the matter, we must look at the first step of quantum creativity described by Dr. Goswami as preparation. The quality of listening and the relationship with the client is essential in achieving an environment that supports the slowing down of the vital body, using the most suitable complementary modalities or technology for the situation.

If you remember the story of my brother, you will remember that the specialist doctors didn't get it right because they quickly concluded that it was a psychosomatic migraine and that my mother was another one of those anxious moms worried about her son. Our family doctor didn't buy this version because he knew my mother and brother. I can remember that he would take the time to come to our home to have tea and be with the family.

Think about how you feel when someone takes the time to listen to one of your complicated situations that you can't figure out by yourself. Sometimes, by just speaking out and feeling completely or unconditionally received in that moment, the solution just pops up. Your friend doesn't have to say much. Without knowing it, you have the answer.

Listening is an art that the medical system today, one based on productivity, can't afford. I can't blame the medical doctor or even the nurses who are under more and more pressure from a bureaucratic and legal practice. Most of the time, for the same or less income, these health-care practitioners have to perform many duties that have nothing to do with the direct care of their patients. The solution is obviously to make more time, but that's easier to say than to perform within an environment not designed for it.

A potential solution will be the subject of the last chapter of this book. Here we are proposing the training of a specific type of practitioner who will be able to provide complementary modalities of healing which require more time, within the existing medical system. We call this practitioner a holistic medical assistant.

Listening is one aspect. Another aspect, which is not any less important, is to slow down the vital body, as Dr. Goswami points out. Creativity will find its way more easily when someone is in a relaxed mode, rather than in a stressed sympathetic mode (dominated by the sympathetic nervous system) where thinking is difficult. This is more often the case when one has to face the verdict of an impressive professional team, often all white coated. To add even more tension to this scenario, the words chosen are not always the carriers of a healing force. The fatality of a diagnosis doesn't have the effect of a placebo. It has more the opposite effect, where the patient has to face a problematic issue.

Creative integrative medicine, in this context, can help by proposing many different modalities with the specific goal of switching the client into a more parasympathetic mode of relaxation. Meditation, quantum biofeedback, and other relaxation techniques such as yoga (certainly a popular one) can be used. Aromatherapy, herbology, naturopathy, and homeopathy can also support the client with different cocktails that can do more than just provide relaxation. In some cases, they can open the mind to creative healing.

You have probably understood by this time that the goal is to create, from the beginning, an environment that will allow for creativity. Listening, relaxing, and being compassionate, human, and personal will create the space for obtaining a new awareness about the dramatic and conflicted situations the client is caught in. In *What the Bleep Do We Know?!* the phenomenon of a person's distortion of reality is well portrayed. Quantum medicine, in decoding the emotional conflict associated with any disease with an emotional component, such as a psychosomatic disease, chronic disease, or cancer, is addressing the same problematic issues. Here, the mind has to collapse a new perception or meaning to replace the previous conflicted events that were consequently translated into specific symptoms within the client's physiology.

Incubation

The second part of the quantum creativity process has been described by Dr. Goswami as the incubation period, where the unconscious comes into play. Everyone has experienced an original idea at least once in their life when they least expected it—either in a moment of silence or after a period of relaxation. History has revealed to us so many of these anecdotal incidents, from Archimedes to Newton, true or false but easily accepted by common sense. For the clinician, what is important to remember is that you can't force the process. This is where the frustration comes from because in the usual model of medicine, things are expected to get fixed just by taking a pill.

Recognizing the entanglement between the healer and the healed is crucial, since the limitations of the doctor/practitioner are one with those of the client/patient. We have already touched on this subject, but the unconscious aspect of the client can be tainted by the limited awareness of the doctor. Not surprisingly, many patients have had to walk away from standard treatments to explore other paths of healing for their own survival. Suzanna Markus, who wrote the book *6 Months to Live 10 Years Later: An Extraordinary Healing Journey* (2007), is a living testimony of a breast cancer survivor who courageously transformed a dramatic event in her own healing journey into the realization of her own full potential of a vital life. She did this while walking away from the conventional path. A common denominator in all of these stories of courageous women is that they truly went on *le chemin le moins fréquenté* (the road less traveled). They had to reinvent their lives after going through a personal growth experience.

Sudden Insight

The third phase of quantum creativity is certainly the most fascinating and has been described as the sudden insight, the ah-ha moment. In practice, there are as many ah-ha experiences as spontaneous healings in the history of medicine. You have already read several such stories in this book, but you should not expect a specific scenario. These are like love stories. Even though you have read many of them, none seem the same, and it is always unique and personal for those who experience it.

So no expectations—it happens when it happens, or if it has to happen. The doctor is not in control of it, nor is the client/patient. The most favorable attitude, and what is revealed in all of these testimonies, is a state of acceptance and appreciation for everything. It doesn't mean resignation; it's more of an active gratefulness for what is and what will happen. There is a moment of creativity that comes with the letting go of it or when surrendering to something greater than me.

> When vital energy movement is similarly unbalanced and the vital blueprint is faulty, it is to leap into the supramental and create a new blueprint of the desired vital function ... (Goswami 2004, 238).

> Waiting for the supramental intelligence to descend and create the same kind of revolution at the feeling level as the creative insight at the mental level, the next effect of the quantum leap, is the coming into existence of new blueprints to help consciousness to rebuild—regenerate the used-diseased organs (Goswami 2004, 243).

Sudden insights come from the supramental. Creative intuitive moments can manifest like grace, leaving the ego on the side and, helped by right attitude and a positive environment, encourage the healer-healed relationship.

One day, one of my dear students, Diane Blackburn, captured this moment when observing the live blood of her client while performing a live blood analysis with a high-resolution microscope. From the point of view of quantum physics, such a phenomenon can't be directly measured since it is an immaterial event. But the question was this: could we observe it indirectly in the blood, the same way Dr. Masaru Emoto (2001) captured different patterns of thought in relation to crystallization patterns of water. Her thesis described this moment of grace.

> As was my custom with every client since I set to capture on video a movement of consciousness mirrored in the blood, I let the video capture run for the length of the consultation, and frankly, I had totally forgotten that it was running. I was totally engaged with Shelby, a client

who was initially not too open to suggestion and didn't really think that she needed any help … The conversation was going on at an easy pace, and both Shelby and I were caught in the flow of the moment. The atmosphere became very relaxed … Everything was just allowed to unfold on its own impulse, and I was not expecting anything to happen with Shelby's blood. In other words I was not trying to make anything happen in the blood.

It is only when both Shelby and I entered this timeless space that the blood suddenly jolted. The Taoist philosophers call this *Wei Wu Wei*, doing by not doing or action without attachment. (Blackburn 2013)

I myself have observed modifications of the morphology of blood in many circumstances when applying different techniques of healing, but I found the observation experiment of Dr. Blackburn regarding a creative instant to be very special.

I believe that these moments of creativity are manifesting themselves more often than we realize. Most of the time, the practitioners, either through lack of attention or by ignoring the phenomenon, don't capitalize on the preciousness of this information. But this isn't the only problem here. Even if a doctor has some knowledge of this event, it may often only signal the beginning of the journey. In some cases, but in my point of view rarely, the event may be so powerful that it will create an instant revolution that will impact the physiology of the individual. However, this is typically just the initial awakening that the practitioner can build upon and help a client with and, through the use of multiple strategies, convert into a definitive healing.

Manifestation

This next step of quantum creativity, manifestation, is described by Dr. Goswami as creating new brain circuits within an individual. Today, this is at the core of an emerging science called neuroplasticity. Dr. Joe Dispenza, another well-known presenter in the movie *What the Bleep Do We Know?!* addresses this issue in his books *Breaking the Habit of Being Yourself* (2012) and *Evolve Your Brain* (2007), and now through Quantum University's online brain and neuroplasticity course (2013).

Mind-based medicine is yet another way to describe this large field of interest, and without question, it should be taught to the modern doctor, as we are doing at Quantum University. Other approaches demonstrating successful results include neurolinguistic programming (NLP), meditation, and visualization, which have all been used to anchor what I call definitive healing.

The step of manifestation focuses even more on the client/patient taking an active role, meaning that along with the process, the new awareness produced by a sudden or progressive awakening will bring changes in habits of all types—from thinking to eating. This is often the painful part of the equation. Who wants to listen to it?

In the midst of my medical practice in Canada, I was exposed to all types of desperate situations and sometimes had to weigh in on how motivated the individual was to accept new habits of behavior. I would ask, "Have you had enough of this problem? Are you ready to let go of anything to see this situation disappear?" Surprisingly, the answer was not always affirmative. I realized that we usually would prefer to have it both ways or even die rather than let go of deep-rooted emotions. I also discovered that more advanced strategies were necessary to support the client moving toward personal growth. The old-fashioned way, where the doctor tries to shake up their client, has not worked for a long time.

To demonstrate the importance of the manifestation stage, let's bring back the patient and friend I spoke about at the beginning of the book, Paul Remy. As you could see by his medical condition, he was a living medical encyclopedia. And on the top of all the problems I described previously, he was also a type II diabetic. One day he came for his regular follow-up visit and shared with me that on the previous Sunday, when he was listening to one of his regular religious TV programs, he felt a chill all over his body. There is even more to that story, as he then told me that he should stop his medications for diabetes, since he had the conviction that they were no longer necessary. I obviously discouraged him from doing so and said we should check his blood sugar first. As a result of the tests, it wasn't too long afterward that I agreed to follow his first intuition. But this is still not the end of the story.

Months later, I paid him a home visit. Paul Remy amicably offered me a soft drink. Okay … But I had to go to the basement to get one since he was short of these in his fridge. I went downstairs and found a big reserve of them. "What is this?" I asked him. I hadn't realized that my friend/patient hadn't modified his eating habits and was relying solely on the grace of God. Obviously, later on, the previous condition of diabetes came back. I was at the beginning of my understanding of these types of events then and was still missing a lot of privileged information that has since been refined in quantum medicine today.

Opening the Door to Spontaneous Healings

Star Wars movies have fascinated more than a generation of viewers over the past thirty years, illustrating a fictional universe that mixes philosophy, religion, and futuristic technology in a world where many creatures, half-human and half-reptile or humanoid, live. "May the force be with you" has since imprinted the collective mind and leaves with us a hope that the "dark side" can be conquered by the power of the good. What also amazingly captured our imagination was to witness that there could be a force within, taught by apparently the most vulnerable one, Yoda, which could be learned about and mastered.

Quantum medicine is in some ways the expression of a similar philosophy, one that conveys that the power of healing is within and can be understood through quantum physics and mastered by healers, practitioners, and doctors. The perception of medicine has shifted from a linear, materialistic model to a model of full potential. In this new model, the client/patient can't be caught in the fatalistic reality of a diagnosis, because in this new vision of reality, there is always the possibility of the impossible, as described in spontaneous healings.

The dark side of medicine today is inherent in the consequence of the human body being perceived as a mechanistic model, wherein the genes determine what lies at the end of the road. The dark side of medicine is in denying alternative methods of healing through models of subtle energy. The dark side is to believe in the fatality of a diagnosis or in your genes as a determinant in the equation of healing instead of considering the full potential that exists within the human being.

Colleges of natural medicine and medical universities must embrace the bright side of the knowledge brought forth by quantum physics, which reveals that beyond matter is a fundamental and transcendent reality of infinite possibilities. The modern doctor, as well as any individual motivated to reach their full potential, should be educated and trained in how to tackle this spontaneous power of healing within.

Spontaneous healing is the result of a synchronicity of events that conjugates multiple layers of information. The medicine of the future will be able to acknowledge, through science and technology, the ability to tap into the infinite possibilities brought forth through quantum medicine.

Chapter 3
Integrating Taoist Medicine into a Quantum Model

This chapter is probably one of the most fascinating in the book. Here you will be introduced to the quantum model that will allow you to understand the movement of subtle energy in relation to the morphogenetic field and the organs and meridians associated with it.

Why this so important? Because gaining an understanding of the relationship among the vital body, the mind, and the supramental levels is at the core of mind-based medicine. Without this information, it is almost impossible to translate the human being in terms of potential, a process of personal growth that takes place in which positive health is not just an absence of disease but is also a state of greater personal integration.

Before I go into details, let me share with you another amazing moment in my quest that happened less than twenty years ago. An acupuncturist friend of mine spoke to me one day about a lady from France who was teaching medical astrology. "Please, this is the last thing I would investigate," I told her. I had already trained in homeopathy and acupuncture at that time, but my friend insisted that I at least see her, if only to satisfy my own curiosity. I couldn't resist, even though I couldn't rationalize why I should meet her.

Our first meeting blew my mind completely regarding the personal information she accessed in such a short time. Her understanding was profound and pertinent. Actually, I realize today that her knowledge had nothing to do with astrology; it was more from what I would define as consciousness medicine—a science of the movement of consciousness within and without the individual as micro-cosmos and macro-cosmos. With quantum physics today, it is no longer a stretch to understand that we are not islands but are connected with the whole universe. Not only that, but many scientists are also revealing other dimensions or parallel universes and are even challenging the notion of time.

Her knowledge is represented in the curriculum of Quantum University today as a refinement of the subtle energy anatomy that I presented earlier. My contribution has been to adapt this key information to the context of a quantum model of medicine.

Meeting Marguerite de Surany

So who was this mysterious lady? Her name was Marguerite de Surany. Known in France as a prolific author, she has addressed many subjects including graphology, Yi-King (I-Ching), alchemy, medical astrology, and the psychology of Chinese medicine in relation to spiritual growth. I knew that she had knowledge that I didn't have, even though I had already covered many subjects in complementary medicine. More specifically, she knew how to relate the mechanics of consciousness with imbalances, behavior, organs, and disease, and she introduced me to a new universe wherein acupuncture began to make more sense as she related it to profound information that she called Taoist medicine.

What were her sources? One day after she had published a book on medical graphology, a special group of Taoist doctors noticed her and asked to meet her. She was asked for guidance in the writing of a manuscript concerning the meridians in their relationships with the cosmos and planets. They would guide her in the exactitude of the correlation of her works. This was the beginning of her journey, where she explored the mysteries of the behavior of the soul, entangled with the energetic apparatus of the meridians, their source and origin, and how they are affected by our thoughts, emotions, and conflicts.

I studied under her guidance for two years, and she was one of the greatest mentors of my life. She taught me in great detail what I see today as the internal quantum mechanics of the subtle energy anatomy. She also guided me in my personal spiritual growth and allowed me to understand the dynamics of my own psyche. When I was putting together the masterpieces of the medical curriculum at Quantum University, I couldn't ignore this important and privileged information.

Referring to empiric information, which is the legacy of ancient wisdom, is always a challenge in a context designed to provide information for conventional modern medicine. So the reader has to understand that I share in the Taoist medicine and acupuncture course (Drouin) a small fraction of her deeper *savoir* that can be explained in the context of quantum physics. I apologize to Marguerite today if in some way I have integrated her comprehension into an environment that has to do with quantum physics and medicine. I can hear her voice in the back of my head saying, "Ha! Ca c'est du jolie alors."

A Taoist Subtle Energy Anatomy:
The Rainbow Body, Marvelous Vessels, Kouas, and Meridians

One of her interesting concepts was *"le Corps d'Arc en Ciel"* ("the Rainbow Body") (de Surany 1996). This describes invisible lines called a complex of meridians or avenues of waves, colored by the density of their vibration, and special channels named marvelous vessels, which explain how the original energy flow in the vital body relates with the archetype qualities of the soul. Meridians, connecting to the vital blueprints of organs, sing and express themselves according to the individual mind's reaction to the personal and social events of life, whether joyful or sad, fast or slow, strong or weak shimmering manifestations of changing colors. The result is so luminous that the ancient Tibetan monks called it "the Rainbow Body" (de Surany, *Dictionnaire de Medecine Taoist,* 1996, 85–88).

The Rainbow Body can be seen as a quantic system that allows us to understand the movement of consciousness in the vital body relating to imbalances with the organs, the meridians, and the associated emotions.

This becomes even more sophisticated when we can associate the archetypal value of a higher emotion to another subtle anatomy structure called *Kouas* (de Surany 1996, 85–88), where the meridian gets recharged at different hours of the day. These types of emanations, eight in number, are in some way capital—reservoirs of energy—and are located in the white matter of the spinal cord. Be aware that all of these structures, Kouas or others, are in fact nonlocal—more precisely, nonlocal channels of information related to the spinal cord.

In one instant, these emanations also reflect the qualities of the soul in terms of archetypal emanations, such as

- love-compassion (Chen)
- courage (TaTam)
- wisdom (Roun)
- life force and longevity (Khouen)
- tenacity and tone (Ken)
- capacity of communion (Khan)
- forgiveness (Souen)
- surrendering to the will of God (Sonen)
- high morality (Lo)
- power of manifestation (Khien)

But where do the Kouas originate? Marguerite de Surany would say,

From Emptiness "the Black Hole" is born, a movement "without conception," triggering a fluctuation of infinitesimal quanta, uncontrollable radiation, burning with no possibility of extinction—the Yin-Yang. The One becomes Two: Yang, the principle of light; Yin, the principle of sound. They radiate an uncontrollable burning steam, which envelops them, creating a womb of lead that makes them invisible and inviolable. These radiations collectively bear fruit.

In time and in space, this geyser creates a second womb, formed by a crown of differentiating energies and hierarchies, the *Marvelous Vessels* (de Surany, *le Corps d'Arc en Ciel (The Rainbow Body)* 1996, 143)

From these vessels, the eight emanations condense themselves into eight Kouas. The eight Kouas develop into sixty-four figures of the I-Ching. The sixty-four I-Ching hexagrams, which encode character pattern binary code, are the oldest quantum model. In every figure is encrypted the origin of imbalance and the wisdom to solve it.

The Atomic Heart: A Quantum Model for the Soul

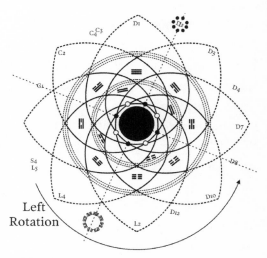

Left Rotation

Figure 3.1: The Atomic Heart
(Quantum Taoist Medicine and Acupuncture Course)

To go deeper, marvelous vessels are nonlocal channels of information that move along the spinal cord and act as filter, captor, regulator, equilibrator, distributor, producer, or the original spark of the original energy. Why is this so meaningful for a consciousness medicine? Because this information is an essential complement of the knowledge of subtle anatomy regarding the vital, mental, supramental, and bliss bodies and also opens the possibility for exploring how to translate health in terms of a higher self-integration.

A Quantum Approach

Let me ask you a question. What is the point of replacing the liver of an alcoholic who will continue to choose a mode of life that will just perpetuate the same habit that destroyed his liver in the first place? In quantum medicine, the symptom or the disease is seen as an alarm for that person to consider some modification of their habits and ways of thinking, leading to healing that comes with a new awareness that guides the individual to new choices, resulting in a higher integration of the self. The Rainbow Body and its apparatus provide a map that allows us to understand more deeply what is going on and also opens a window to act at a more subtle level with different modalities of energetic therapies.

To be healthy is not just about not having a liver disease; rather, it is also about reaching the full potential of what the liver apparatus represents: organ, meridian, Kouas, and marvelous vessels. It is also about having a greater wisdom about life, a better perspective on adjusting personal choices to align with a greater reality of life, and a higher quality of emotion associated with the liver.

Practitioners usually associate the liver with anger or frustration, which is the negative quality of an ego functioning in survival mode. Frustration and anger when things don't happen as we wish is opposite to the positive quality of the soul being aligned with a deeper vision, in resonance with the purpose of the universe, guided by the wisdom to seek a path of lesser resistance more in accordance with divine will. The archetypal essence of wisdom could be related to the nonlocal structure of the Kouas. Keep in mind that according to Dr. Goswami, the supramental is a nonlocal reality.

Remember this image when you are in pain: your energetic structure is shrinking, contracting on itself in a mode of survival, and this will translate in your behavior as a more egoistic reaction. Oppositely, when you are more in a mode of creativity, the energy will flow more freely, expressing a higher quality of the self. These events will then be translated in the vital body, according to a subtle anatomy that has already been perceived for hundreds of years and transmitted through a lineage of great Taoist masters, the masters with whom Marguerite de Surany had the opportunity to work.

Here the individual is the artisan of their own world and imbalance. Through a process of awakening, they will progressively attune with their own divine source and recreate a state of positive health. The Taoist masters revealed that as the individual attunes progressively with higher self qualities, then the Rainbow Body will become as "luminous as the rainbow"—words describing the state of positive health as full potential.

> One day, when every meridian of the Rainbow Body is in perfect harmony with the model offered by the eight Kouas, then the physical body will never fall ill, and the blood will sing in all the vessels of the body (de Surany 1996, 143).

Consciousness Acupuncture

This is why I found it essential to teach about an acupuncture that is more than just a series of protocols for where to puncture for different types of pathologies, more what I call a consciousness acupuncture that explores the real source of a problem. I also introduce the concept of intelligent pathways, which are the marvelous vessels, according to Marguerite de Surany, and related to the Kouas and the meridians, which give access to a more efficient level of information to restore balance and harmony of the morphogenetic field.

These (nonlocal) pathways are found in the ancient scripts of Su Wen, Ling Shu, Nan Jing, and numerous others. Marguerite De Surany compares them to a fiber optic technology where the laser is the meridian and the fiber is the marvelous vessels. Around the central canal and in the gray matter and the cerebral fluid, they move up and down in a spiral. They capture, produce, filter, equilibrate, and distribute, creating an impenetrable wall that protects the nucleus of the creation for which they are the crown.

Kouas radiate in quantity and quality according to the functioning of the marvelous vessels and the energy they receive from ancestral energy. The ability to recharge the meridians from these emanations (Kouas) is related to qualities of the soul.

Here we are using a quantum language to describe how negative emotions or feelings move the subtle morphogenetic fields and manifest illnesses in the physical body. This is something that we already know in another language (e.g., "Your anger may make you sick."). This quantum language can also express how positive emotions or feelings can manifest a higher degree of integration of the morphogenetic fields that allows you to say, "I feel at my best today, as though I am ageless."

The Role of the Creative Integrative Doctor

The challenge for a consciousness-based medicine is to integrate the notion of personal growth, where the individual shifts from functioning in an ego self-centered mode to a more self-universal mode. This is a model of healing where the role of an integrative doctor will be to facilitate the transcendence of the ego-character to the emergence of the quantum self, while keeping in mind that the nature of this conditioned movement is also an energetic one (chi) at the organ, meridian, marvelous vessel, and Koua levels. In addition, the associated conditioned feelings, conditioned emotions, and conditioned movements of the mind (habit patterns) occur.

See the example below of the heart and emotions related to the heart meridian.

Heart: Balance-Excess-Empty

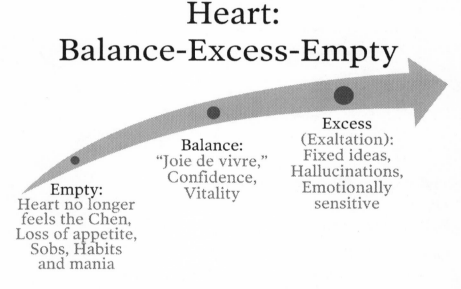

Excess (Exaltation): Fixed ideas, Hallucinations, Emotionally sensitive

Balance: "Joie de vivre," Confidence, Vitality

Empty: Heart no longer feels the Chen, Loss of appetite, Sobs, Habits and mania

**Figure 3.2: The Heart and Emotions
(Quantum Taoist Medicine and Acupuncture Course)**

To do this, the integrative doctor is engaging the creative process simultaneously at all levels of anatomy: the bliss, supramental, mental, vital, and physical bodies. Every level is a reflection of a different quality of information—the bliss being the more subtle and the physical the more solid. Therapies given at a spiritual level can permeate the lower ones, but those given at the lower ones cannot affect the higher ones.

Vital Body Medicine

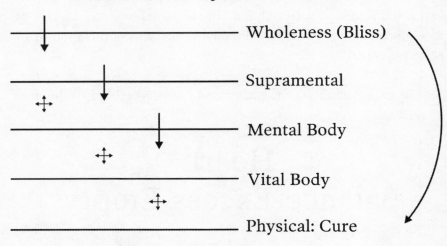

Wholeness (Bliss)

Supramental

Mental Body

Vital Body

Physical: Cure

Figure 3.3: Vital Body Medicine
(Quantum Taoist Medicine and Acupuncture Course)

The Notion of Balance Is Important:
Living in the Ego and Living in the Quantum Self Must Be Balanced in a Life Focused on Spiritual Growth

Quantum medicine proposes an integrative approach that will restore the morphogenetic field, the blueprint for the organs, to its full potential, tuning into a creative mode of operating in relation with the higher self. Positive health is achieved when the physical, vital, mental, supramental, and bliss bodies are in tune and in congruence with the core source.

This is also a foundation for a real preventive medicine, which focuses on subtle energetic imbalances, to be adjusted through the knowledge of a more refined "consciousness acupuncture," involving energetic therapy as well as mind-body approaches. In the decades to come, we will witness the emergence of a new generation of assessment protocols with energetic devices that will help the integrative doctor to prevent disease at a much earlier stage, even when it is still in its thought form state.

Positive Health is expressed when the Physical-Vital-Mental-Supramental are in tune, in congruence with the core source.

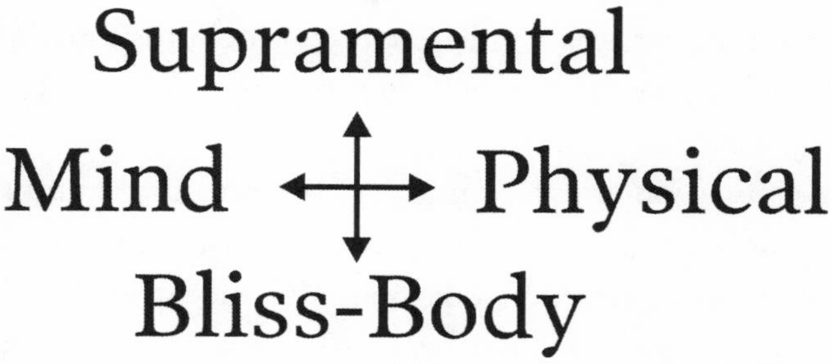

Supramental

Mind ←┼→ Physical

Bliss-Body

Figure 3.4: Positive Health is expressed when the Physical-Vital-Mental-Supramental are in tune. (Quantum Taoist Medicine and Acupuncture Course)

Using the Five Elements to Evaluate a Client

If the marvelous vessels are (nonlocal) intelligent pathways restoring balance, the five elements are a source of strategic information for understanding in more detail the dynamics of emotions and their meaning in regard to the five seasons.

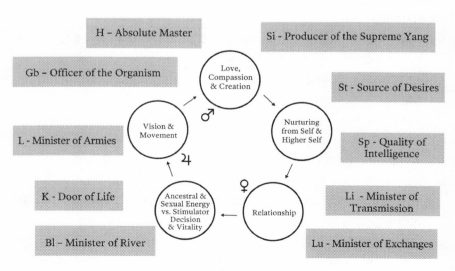

Figure 3.5: The Five Elements
(Quantum Taoist Medicine and Acupuncture Course)

The Taoist tradition is very rich here with information to refine our understanding of the connection between mind and body and to resolve conflict with a deeper understanding. The acupuncture and Taoist medicine course I created is unique in the sense that this material is revealed for the first time in the context of quantum medicine and is distinguished from conventional acupuncture.

To make evaluation simpler and to create an understanding of how emotions and thoughts can influence organs, meridians, Kouas, and marvelous vessels, I created a questionnaire with questions that reflect the mode of how the individual reacts to life, scaled to assess subjectively the level of their integration.

For example, for the heart, one of the five elements (that can also be related to the heart chakra), the questions formulated would be the following:

How is your fire?
Did you grow up in a warm family?
Was it a cold family relationship?
Hardhearted?
Have you been brokenhearted more than twice in your life?
Are joy and laughter in your life?
Are friendships important to you?
Are you often depressed?
How easy is it for you to give?
How easy is it for you to receive?
What was the relationship between your father and mother?
Do you feel that you were loved in your childhood?
In relationships, are you concerned about the happiness of your partner?
Do you accept yourself?
If you had the possibility of changing your appearance, would you?
Is it easier to accept yourself when someone appreciates you?

You can see in the diagram below that the meridian will be in insufficiency (at the extreme empty), balanced, or in excess, with possible associated symptoms.

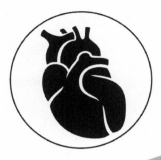

Heart
(Physical)

Insufficiency/Empty - Balance - Excess

Bright
eyes,
Vitality

Too much
sonority in
the voice,
Quick laugh

Painful
heart,
Palpitations

Figure 3.6: Heart Meridian (Physical)
(Quantum Taoist Medicine and Acupuncture Course)

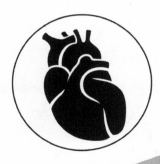

Heart
(Vital-Mental)

Insufficiency/Empty - Balance - Excess

"Joie de vivre,"
Confidence,
Vitality

Fixed ideas,
Hallucinations,
Sensitive
emotionally

Heart no
longer feels the
Chen, Loss of Appetite,
Sobs, Habits, Mania

Figure 3.7: Heart Meridian (Vital–Mental)
(Quantum Taoist Medicine and Acupuncture Course)

The same scenario can be applied through the five elements approach using the kidney meridian.

How is your vital energy?
When you wake up in the morning, are you full of energy?
Do you tend to feel tired all the time?
Do you take time during the day to reenergize yourself?
Do you feel drained all the time, as though you don't have enough time to accomplish what you have to do?
Are you often insecure?
Are you anxious about the future?
How is your sex life?
Is it difficult for you make decisions?
Do you feel overwhelmed by situations?
Do you feel sleepy all the time?
Are you bitter about life?
Do you always want more?
Do you feel so discouraged that you feel you just don't have the will to face another day?

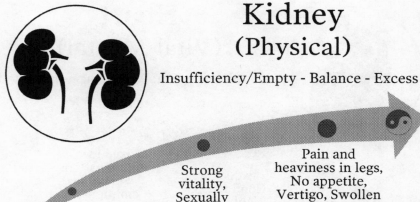

Kidney
(Physical)
Insufficiency/Empty - Balance - Excess

Strong vitality, Sexually vital

Pain and heaviness in legs, No appetite, Vertigo, Swollen eyes, Difficulty in hearing, Sore throat

Low back pain, Frequent urination, Impotence, Deafness

Figure 3.8: Kidney Meridian (Physical)
(Quantum Taoist Medicine and Acupuncture Course)

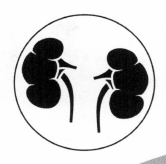

Kidney
(Vital-Mental)

Insufficiency/Empty - Balance - Excess

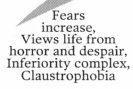

Authoritarian,
Exaggerated
vitality, Ruse,
Restlessness

Strong
character,
Sharp intelligence,
Sexually vital,
Considerable
will, Strong
vitality

Fears
increase,
Views life from
horror and despair,
Inferiority complex,
Claustrophobia

Figure 3.9: Kidney Meridian (Vital–Mental)
(Quantum Taoist Medicine and Acupuncture Course)

Keep in mind that these questions are not exhaustive, but they are clues that will guide the practitioner to understand what's going on and to correlate with the client what can help them reach a greater awareness of the drama they are caught in, which may help to trigger ah-ha moments, as described in the quantum creativity chapter (chapter 2).

This methodology also provides the integrative doctor with a way to access the energetic paths that can shift the situation of the client. The work could also be done using any type of vital energy therapy approach, from acupuncture to homeopathy, to shake the level of energy where the unbalanced situation is frozen. Breathing, yoga, or other mind-body techniques can melt the state of fear or lack of fire where the client is stuck.

Quantum medicine opens the door to creativity and makes available other modalities of healing. When the quantum practitioner understands the map of the mechanics for healing, all possibilities become available to them.

Chakra Medicine

While the Taoist and Chinese medicine traditions have brought to us the knowledge of meridians, Ayurvedic medicine is more familiar with the notion of chakras. Chakra means "wheel" in Sanskrit. Dr. Goswami would say, "Feelings are the experience of the chakra's vital energy—the movements of your morphogenetic fields, which are correlated with the organs of which they are the blueprint/source." A classic example is to ask, "Where do you feel love?" Everyone points to the area of the heart chakra.

Chakras have been associated though different traditions with a variety of qualities and functions.

Organs, Glands, Chakras, Dominant Feelings

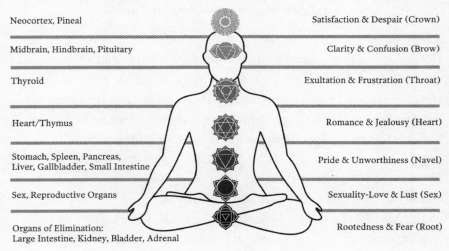

Neocortex, Pineal	Satisfaction & Despair (Crown)
Midbrain, Hindbrain, Pituitary	Clarity & Confusion (Brow)
Thyroid	Exultation & Frustration (Throat)
Heart/Thymus	Romance & Jealousy (Heart)
Stomach, Spleen, Pancreas, Liver, Gallbladder, Small Intestine	Pride & Unworthiness (Navel)
Sex, Reproductive Organs	Sexuality-Love & Lust (Sex)
Organs of Elimination: Large Intestine, Kidney, Bladder, Adrenal	Rootedness & Fear (Root)

Figure 3.10: Chakra associations with organs, glands and dominant feelings (Quantum Hormonology Course)

Sometimes, there are variations in these correlations. Marguerite de Surany agreed that they belong to the Indian tradition and are located in the gray matter of the spinal cord.

Again, you have to understand that chakras, like meridians, are nonlocal and are another dimensional layer of information associated with these locations. Chakras get their intensity through the quality of the marvelous vessels (and Kouas), resonating from the ancestral energy where they originate. She doesn't suggest approaching them directly through acupuncture.

Interestingly, we can also relate these nonlocal structures to glands and nerve plexuses in our anatomy. This fact makes them more attractive to conventional medicine, of course, since there is something more tangible to refer to.

I like to look at them as transformative *athanor*. In alchemy, an athanor is a furnace used to provide a uniform and constant heat for alchemical digestion. In this case, one can experience not only feelings but also provide access by reason of their complex correlations (with organs, meridians, Kouas, marvelous vessels, associated glands, function, and purpose), through a variety of energetic work including meditation, breathing, and other vital body approaches.

Chakras & Vital Body Functions, Organs, & Glands

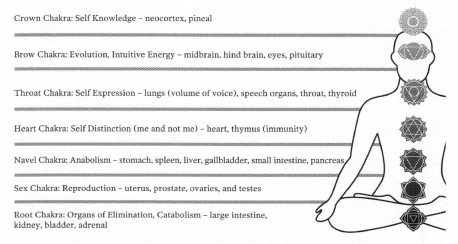

Crown Chakra: Self Knowledge – neocortex, pineal

Brow Chakra: Evolution, Intuitive Energy – midbrain, hind brain, eyes, pituitary

Throat Chakra: Self Expression – lungs (volume of voice), speech organs, throat, thyroid

Heart Chakra: Self Distinction (me and not me) – heart, thymus (immunity)

Navel Chakra: Anabolism – stomach, spleen, liver, gallbladder, small intestine, pancreas

Sex Chakra: Reproduction – uterus, prostate, ovaries, and testes

Root Chakra: Organs of Elimination, Catabolism – large intestine, kidney, bladder, adrenal

Figure 3.11: Chakras and vital body functions, organs, and glands (Quantum Hormonology Course)

The original research of Dr. Joe Dispenza on brain neuroplasticity implements a vital bodywork using meditation and breathing techniques focusing on the chakras to create new brain circuits associated with healing. The results are astonishing and have been documented with brain mapping. This is discussed in detail in the class taught by Dr. Dispenza in our curriculum and is complemented by Dr. Jeffrey Fanning, who was responsible for the scientific research (Dispenza 2013).

The chakras can be also an interesting source of information during the process of evaluating the level of integration of the individual.

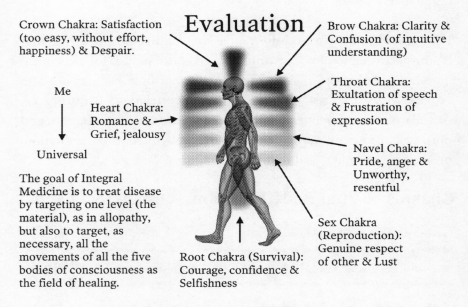

Evaluation

Crown Chakra: Satisfaction (too easy, without effort, happiness) & Despair.

Brow Chakra: Clarity & Confusion (of intuitive understanding)

Throat Chakra: Exultation of speech & Frustration of expression

Me

Heart Chakra: Romance & Grief, jealousy

Universal

Navel Chakra: Pride, anger & Unworthy, resentful

The goal of Integral Medicine is to treat disease by targeting one level (the material), as in allopathy, but also to target, as necessary, all the movements of all the five bodies of consciousness as the field of healing.

Root Chakra (Survival): Courage, confidence & Selfishness

Sex Chakra (Reproduction): Genuine respect of other & Lust

Figure 3.12: Evaluating the level of integration using the Chakras (Quantum Hormonology Course)

The movement of consciousness from the root chakra to the crown chakra will be imprinted into qualities of the quantum self, as seen in the previous graphic, and will provide clues for the integrative doctor to subjectively perform their evaluation. Chakra medicine, as quantum medicine, is also about the full potential of the representation of the function of the chakras.

The heart chakra is an easy example of this concept. The more the client is in an ego mode, the more qualities like possessiveness, fear of loss, grief, hurt, and jealousy will be expressed, compared to the higher self mode, where one will be more in a state of compassion and universal love.

Chapter 4
Quantum Homeopathy

Homeopathy is a model of healing that is very well suited to quantum physics—a science that explores the infinitesimal reality of the universe. While numerous studies have proven the therapeutic efficacy of many homeopathic products in clinics, the medical establishment is still not enthusiastic about bringing homeopathy back inside its walls. In fact, in 1900 there were twenty-two homeopathic colleges and 15,000 practitioners in the United States, and homeopathy was considered an official medicine (Toufexis 1995). Obviously, for many reasons, the status of homeopathy is no longer the same. From my point of view, the best strategy for bringing it back will be to lay out a new foundation of understanding for this medicine based on premises that will appear valid to a scientific and reasonable mind.

Samuel Hahnemann described homeopathy in his book *The Organon of the Healing Art* (1833), known as the bible of homeopathy, as a "spirit-like" force that sustains and maintains life and as the vital force that produces the symptoms in its effort to rid the body of disease. But he was not preparing for the acceptance of homeopathy by the materialistic twentieth-century community. His vision had to wait for the twenty-first century, where a new understanding of the universe can now make sense out of eleventh centesimal dilution, in which there is no longer any of the original substance remaining in the homeopathic preparation.

The Vital Force

Understanding the function of the vital force is one of the cornerstones of homeopathy. The vital force is responsible for maintaining the body in a balanced state of health.

> The Vital Force is not enclosed in man, but radiates around him like a luminous sphere, and it may be made to act at distance. Through these rays of subtle form, the imagination of man may produce healthy or morbid effects. (*The Life and the Doctrines of Paracelsus,* Hartman)

This was the language of that time in history. Today, with the principles of quantum physics, we can make sense of it. Through the model of a subtle energy anatomy, we can understand that the vital body is the layer of information that can be associated with the vital force. This underlying reality is nonlocal and can explain why beyond the eleventh centesimal dilution, where there is apparently no more measurable substance, consciousness then becomes the mediator of this information. It also explains why intention and the entanglement between healer and the healed can influence the outcome of the therapy.

The vital body refers to this layer of information where the vital movements associated with thoughts and feelings create a specific energetic signature that individualizes our specific history of conditioning. When the vital movements go wrong, causing disease at the physical level, there must be a corresponding energetic signature to the vital energy imbalance. The vital body becomes the mirror of the physical body.

Homeopathy is a repertory of energetic signatures that have been manufactured through a subtle process of diluting and energizing (a process called succussion) substances including plants, minerals, etc. Homeopathy offers the possibility of correcting these vital body imbalances by identifying the vital energy signature of the particular medicinal substance that resonates the best with the unbalanced vital energy signature of the individual client.

My Clinical Experiences Integrating Homeopathy

As I described in the introduction, I came to homeopathy because of the frustration I was having with antibiotic therapy, especially in young children during the long and cold winters in Canada. I felt that I was weakening them through the repetitive use of antibiotics, whereas with homeopathy I could make them more resistant to infection by strengthening their bioterrain and constitution. For peace of mind, I added a tympanometry device to my practice. You seldom find this in a family doctor's practice. It is typically a test done by an otorhinolaryngology specialist. With this test, I could measure more precisely the condition of the middle ear and the mobility of the eardrum (tympanic membrane) by creating variations of air pressure in the ear canal. This objective test confirmed to me that the homeopathic approach was successful and without side effects with young patients. At that time, I ran a successful home study with at least fifty cases, which I later presented in the context of a homeopathic conference.

In the chapter on quantum creativity (chapter 2), I described how a patient who was not responding to conventional therapies for a critical condition and who was at risk for amputation of his leg was rescued by homeopathy. In reality, the one who heals is not always "right." In conventional medicine, healing is not the only goal because procedures must be done according to the standards defined by the medical mainstream. One day, one of my colleagues had to face the disciplinary committee of the medical board because he had prescribed a homeopathic substance to his client who was cured of a thyroid condition. The question was not whether the patient was cured or not but rather that an "illegitimate" substance was used to treat his patient.

Fortunately, I was able to practice homeopathy for many years, as the medical board was more tolerant in my case. In the beginning, I implemented homeopathy on a very small scale, essentially for children. As I became more knowledgeable with this model of healing, my practice expanded to a broader range of patients. My prescriptions at the beginning of my practice as a general practitioner were 100 percent pharmaceutical. After ten years, this shifted to 95 percent natural-based prescriptions, with the majority based on homeopathy. I had to deal with very complicated cases, where most clients had already consulted specialists without any resolution for their health problems before they came to see me.

Patients came from all parts of Canada, and some even came from the United States. I treated a whole spectrum of diseases including chronic diseases such as chronic fatigue syndrome, autoimmune disease, allergies, and cancer, to name a few. All of these clients were brought to my office by word of mouth. If I could help one client that couldn't find a solution after having exhausted all other official means of healing, this inevitably brought me ten more. I did not have the pretension that I could cure everything, but I could certainly provide ease to everyone.

My understanding that all modalities of healing could be integrated for the best outcome for the patient was very successful. Homeopathy was an important adjunct in this perspective because it addressed the individual more from the root cause. I would never discourage the patient from a pharmaceutical medication when it was necessary, but I would not overuse it in order to avoid all the side effects associated with it. Modern medicine should take greater advantage of this approach. Through a pluralistic homeopathic approach, I added another important branch of homeopathy—homotoxicology—which has a profound effect on a client's bioterrain. I won't go in depth in this book as to how these modalities were implemented, but I have a firm conviction that this science of healing should be an important component of the curriculum of traditional or natural medicine training, such as we have at our university.

I still have in mind many client stories that can support my position. Seasonal allergies brought many clients to my clinic. One day, a very interesting lady with allergies and chronic migraines finally found her solution for these conditions that had been bothering her for many years. This story became more interesting when she shared with me that her horse had a chronic cough that no veterinarian could alleviate. From the beginning, I tried to avoid the case, but she was so insistent that I finally suggested a homeopathic remedy for her special pet. The result was almost instantaneous. She was so excited by the outcome that she gave me a picture of the horse that I proudly kept on my desk. Meanwhile, she convinced one of her veterinarians to become a homeopath, to my grand satisfaction, since I could not keep up with this growing equine clientele.

Later on, as happened every year, I had a visit from a representative of my medical board. To keep an eye on my "deviant" practice, he would randomly look at my patient files to see if I was still respecting the basic principles of conventional medicine. Year after year, he would make a few recommendations, all the while satisfied that I kept my patients well documented and evaluated according to the strict standards of medicine. I also took care to be the first private office to become computerized, so the data for the clients was transparent and easily accessible.

When doing this evaluation, he sat at my desk like he owned the place. This was very intimidating. Then the horse picture caught his attention, so he didn't hesitate to investigate more. I thought he would be impressed by the story and perhaps be convinced that homeopathy was not just a placebo. He listened very attentively, keeping his reaction for the end. As he left my home office, I can remember him in the doorway laughing and saying, "By the way, the story about the horse, this is a good one!"

A family doctor is exposed to many kinds of clinical situations that most will never find the answer for in a medical textbook. For many of these unusual situations, the conventional doctor doesn't have a resolution and many will label them as "This is in your head" or "It's psychosomatic." Or some will say, "Consult me again if it becomes more serious." How many of you have seen your generalist for something strange, and after the doctor has touched the suspected area of your body, you'll be told, "Oh, this is nothing." You are not really reassured, but what can you do except to get used to it, if you don't want be looked at as "crazy" or weird?

A lady who was a professional psychologist didn't give up, probably because she was more confident about her sanity. Her problem was quite uncomfortable, since she could not sit for more than a half hour without having to go to the bathroom. Men of a certain age can understand this situation. In her case, after she went through all the routine tests including a cystoscopy, nobody could give her comfort for her situation. When she saw me for the first visit, she even had to excuse herself since she couldn't go through the whole consultation without needing the bathroom. Telling her that this was in her head was not an option. I complemented her evaluation with the type of investigation discussed in the chapter on patient evaluation (chapter 6). Her case was easily solved with a specific diet and a homeopathic remedy to calm her urge to urinate. I also had a lot of success with men, post-prostatectomy, who were experiencing a persistent irritation without any sign of infection. Chronic headaches after brain trauma, common migraines, and tension headaches also respond very well to homeopathy.

In the popular mind, the general thinking is that doctors and health professionals disregard the systematic use of homeopathy. You may be amazed that the same percentage of professionals who are interested in natural medicine in all of its forms also believe this more so than the general population. I advised many health professionals in my practice for their personal use too. One major reason that motivated them to come to me was that they didn't want to take the medications they were prescribing for their patients because of the side effects. Of course, when they improved, the classic answer "I don't know if this was you" suggested that their condition had disappeared, but in a safe way so as to still keep their credibility.

I could continue on and on, story after story, and still not convince the skeptic looking for more proof than even standard medical practitioners had when important new therapies over the past thirty years were first introduced. If you have any doubt, I invite you to survey the use of hormone therapy with women. You will discover that the experiments most often happened in the field, where doctors readjusted dosages and combinations of different hormones in response to dangerous side effects encountered. Two to three years ago, I received a notice from my medical board condemning the use of one of the most common hormonal prescriptions for menopause that had been in use since I started my medical practice.

I never had side effects with the use of homeopathy, except for mild symptoms of detoxification that are easily predictable with proper training. This medicine has to be taken seriously and should be in the hands of properly trained professionals. Too often, the fact that homeopathy is not associated with side effects means that it is used by weekend practitioners. It doesn't mean that we should not educate people on the basic use of homeopathy for the family, but putting these very powerful modalities in the hands of incompetent practitioners is also questionable.

In a few years, as I said earlier, homeopathy and homotoxicology will be as important as pharmacology in the curriculum of study for the creative integrative doctor.

Research of Homeopathic Applications

The model of research used for homeopathy needs to be completely redefined within the new parameters provided by quantum physics. The linear model of research isn't comprehensive enough to understand the mechanics of most of the systems of healing based on subtle energy. Quantum physics acknowledges many phenomena that can't be understood by the standard linear scientific model, such as these:

- Thoughts are not local and can have an effect at a distance and can either heal or create imbalance.

- Positive health is embedded within everyone in the quantum self.

- Health is expressed in terms of a potential that can be actualized through proper knowledge and tuning.

This language is more suitable within the context of quantum physics, and it will support thousands of research studies already done and rejected because a linear model of science could not grasp the subtlety of this healing reality.

When Jacques Benveniste published his controversial paper in 1988 in the scientific journal *Nature*, the materialistic scientific community at that time was obviously not ready for this model of understanding. But in 2013, the concept of the memory of water has found many supporters all over the world, respectable scientists among them.

This is one of the main points of this book, to bring attention to a new scientific perspective in medicine that at this time is emerging and is now part of creative integrative medicine.

Chapter 5
Quantum Hematology

This chapter will discuss one of the most important dogmas in medicine concerning the blood and how we look at it. Hematology will be viewed from the perspective of quantum physics, what I call today quantum hematology. This represents the beginning of an understanding and integration of knowledge about blood microscopy that has been put aside for many years, simply because it did not fit within a linear protocol of looking at the most precious tissue in the body: the blood. Most medical doctors today have no idea that many years ago, the decision to look at this precious tissue would have tremendous consequences for the future of medicine. Once again, how we look at things matters.

Hundreds of years of observing the morphology of the blood with dark field and phase contrast microscopy has supplied us with incalculable knowledge regarding what we call the *milieu interieur* of the body— or in an even more poetic language, the *mirror of the soul.* Today, many doctors indoctrinated in the traditional Western scientific model of medicine disregard years of documented experiences of clinical correlations with the blood for the simple reason that it is not taught in medical schools.

Creative integrative medicine is about to create an environment where many types of medicine can be at the service of the sick and the weak. It will also be a system where any parameters necessary can be used to shift from the obsessive search for a fatal diagnosis toward a deeper understanding of the real cause of the problems. By doing so, the reader may realize that we are simultaneously shaking the foundations of the whole business of medicine.

Do we need still more studies to support the concept of quantum hematology? Probably, but there is already a lot of information about hematology that we can look at, considering that it has been helpful in treating thousands of individuals on a clinical basis in natural medicine. Keep in mind that the experiments that we will discuss in this chapter are reproducible at very low cost and can make sense to a rational mind only if you consider this new foundation for viewing blood: "hematology within consciousness."

Integrating Bechamp and Pasteur Theories

The historic dispute between Bechamp and Pasteur regarding the question of germs as the cause of disease is legendary, even though I never heard about it in medical school. Obviously, Pasteur's point of view, best known by medical doctors, was chosen and today serves as the cornerstone of the pharmacologic approach to infections. For over a hundred years, Bechamp's theory that the interior terrain means everything and the microbe nothing has been a well-kept secret in the backyards of alternative medicine.

In conventional hematology, based on the Pasteur point of view, blood is sterile and antibiotics are the therapeutic arsenal used to handle the situation if there are invaders. "Not so fast," said Bechamp. Based on years of observation, this *milieu interieur* can also be influenced by many factors, including the patient's diet, stress level, or emotional state, to name a few. This bioterrain can also be the milieu for degenerative morphologic forms to be observed.

Nobody doubts that the antibiotic therapies developed as a result of Pasteur's germ theory have saved millions of lives, nor can antibiotics be disqualified solely on the basis of the undesirable side effects associated with them. On the other hand, in the tenants of the theory that focuses on the bioterrain where the internal milieu is considered the key to improving immunity and preventing infections, you will see as much conviction about the importance of this point of view. It is amazing what a simple drop of blood can reveal about an individual, in terms of nutritional needs, immune status, and even more, as we will see.

Why should one perspective disqualify the other one? Can we not approach it from an angle where both views could be integrated? This is what is being proposed in quantum hematology: a scientific foundation for hematology based on quantum physics that can integrate both theories.

Medical doctors may have a hard time accepting that you can look at the blood not only in quantitative terms but also from a qualitative perspective. But in doing so, they are missing a big piece of the whole picture. You can't tell me that the qualitative evaluation of patients, providing information about their physical traits and appearance, is not just as important in bringing precious information to the diagnostic process.

Blood Analysis

Having had the privilege of studying at several different schools of blood microscopy, I have realized that a rigid consensus regarding the reading of the blood does not exist. The European school of microscopy rallies more around the idea of *pleomorphism*. (The term comes from the Greek *pleion* for "more" and *morphe* for "form.") Günther Enderlein (1925) became well-known for his concept of the *pleomorphism* of microorganisms and his hypotheses about the origins of cancer, based on the work of other scientists studying the origins of disease at that time. According to Enderlein's theory, the human body lives in symbiosis with primitive life forms called endobionts. Depending on the environment (pH), the protein colloid nature of these forms can evolve in different stages from non-pathogenic to pathogenic (the most advanced are fungi) forms. You can imagine that this theory is a stretch from a conventional viewpoint.

The American schools of live blood analysis have developed a more dietetic approach, leaving aside the idea of pleomorphism, which couldn't be defended in conventional hematology. Bradford and Allen (1997) have done interesting research on oxidative mechanisms with relation to blood coagulation. They have found that free radical activities will create a more soluble clot, triggering characteristic patterns of coagulation, which a simple dry drop of blood on a slide can demonstrate. They look at the blood more as an open echo system that reflects what is going on in the bowel or anywhere else in the physical body itself.

My approach, which I call quantum hematology, is inspired by the principles presented by Dr. Goswami and attempts to reorganize this divergent information from the point of view of having consciousness as its foundation—in other words, *live and dry blood analysis (LBA) with consciousness.* Even if many parameters of live and dry blood analysis could be related to scientific data, especially regarding nutrition, some are still empirical, clinically related, or like pleomorphism, will never suit the conventional model of science.

Quantum hematology, by acknowledging the principles of quantum physics, expands the understanding of the bioterrain to include the vital, mental, supramental, and spiritual energetic bodies as described by Dr. Goswami. These subtle bodies are nonlocal, as explained in Dr. Goswami's book *The Quantum Doctor* when discussing the issue of quantum measurement.

This viewpoint infers that subtle changes in the blood could be indirectly reflecting the activity of the nonlocal energetic bodies as well as the local physical one. The interaction between vital body (as a subtle energy aspect of the bioterrain) and blood (physical aspect of the bioterrain) can be solved by the statement that both are quantum possibilities of consciousness. This applies the same logic used by Dr. Goswami regarding the dichotomy of mind and body. In other words, the blood can indirectly mirror both the physical and subtle energy bioterrain environments.

But can we indirectly assess the activity going on in these subtle layers of information? Isn't an EEG indirectly reflecting if your mind is calm, sleeping, or in activity? Can we indirectly have an idea of what is going on in these subtle compartments of information by observing some qualitative modification of the blood? There is no reason that the morphology of the blood, in regard to its plasticity, could not be interpreted this way.

The work of Dr. Masuru Emoto, which has been popularized by the movie *What the Bleep Do We Know?!* and profusely dispersed on the Web, suggests that our thoughts can affect the structure of the water. As it is possible to observe modification in the crystalline structure of water consequent to different emotional states, the blood can also show the reflection of nonlocal subtle bodies of information. Seeing the unseen reflected in this precious tissue is believing. The advantage that we have with dark field microscopy and live and dry blood analysis is that these experiments are easily reproducible.

Putting It into Practice

Inspired by the many ideas and approaches to blood analysis that I had learned, I decided to incorporate hematology into my own integrative medical practice. Over several years, I observed qualitative modifications of the blood morphology of my clients when viewing it before and after the application of various natural, energetic, and spiritual approaches to healing. Since blood is in major part water, why should we not see a change in its morphologic structure as a significant response? These concepts in hematology and my observations were the subject of a series of conferences in a Seeing Is Believing tour I did throughout Canada and the United States in 2009–2011 (Drouin 2009-2011).

The main idea here, before we go more into detail as to how these experiments were done, is that the blood is much more than a sterile fluid that can only be evaluated in quantitative terms. The blood is an open echo system that reflects the movement of consciousness in physical, vital, mental, and spiritual bioterrains. Without going too deeply into the course on quantum hematology, let me just say that some parameters have been found to be more sensitive than others in indirectly reflecting what is happening in the subtle bodies. The degree of oxidation in the blood that can be easily observed through the coagulation process of a specimen of dry blood (a simple drop of dry blood observed on a slide with bright field at low 4x or 10x) is one of them. Free radicals affecting the coagulation cascade are another. They are reliable not only in assessing the oxidative mechanism but also as an indirect measurement of the subtle bodies. The degenerative alterations of membranes of the red blood cells in live blood are classic observations recognized even in conventional hematology. Activities of the white blood cells associated with an increase of non-pathogenic forms of fungi in the blood are other relevant parameters. The developmental stages (more or less pathogenic, depending on their degree of development of valency) also provide us with an indirect way to monitor vital body activity and a direct way to monitor the physical activity.

In chapter 6 on evaluation, I will talk more about how many parameters in blood morphology can be interpreted as information that can be used to help actualize the full health potential of an individual. The application and integration with the five pillars approach will be presented in more detail as well. Here, the main idea to note is that blood analysis could be used for monitoring the physical terrain as well as what is happening in the unseen in the nonlocal entities, where consciousness is the mediator of information (as described by Goswami). Another interesting phenomena that I discovered through my own observations and research is that the impact of the application of different treatment therapies (whether spiritual, mental, vital, or physically based) could be reflected in the morphology of the blood. The graphic below (figure 5.1) illustrates different therapies and their influence at different layers of information.

Bio-Vital-Mental-Supramental-Spiritual Terrain

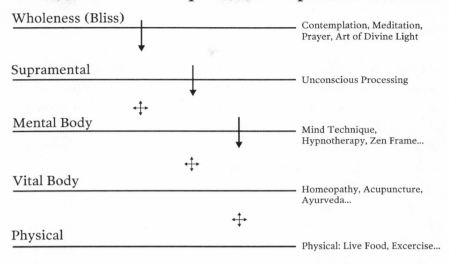

Figure 5.1: The Source of Healing (Quantum Hematology Course)

In other words, what will be observed in the blood—the qualitative morphologic structure of the blood—will represent the indirect energetic signature of a nonlocal activity (bliss-supramental-mental-vital) or of a local activity (physical). (See figure 5.2.)

Template of Signatures

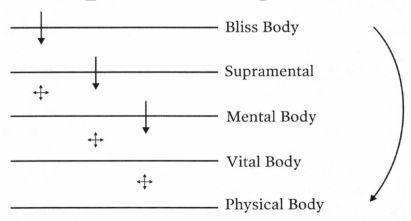

Figure 5.2: The Template of Signatures (Quantum Hematology Course)

Clinical Experiences with Patients

The Effects of Prayer

Let me share with you an amazing clinical experience I had early on in my practice. It will illustrate the example of a spiritual event that demonstrates that prayers can absolutely change the infrastructure of the blood. After the apparent spontaneous healing of Paul Remy through a group prayer (mentioned in chapter 1), I prepared myself to be better equipped for the next unforeseen event.

I had recently incorporated a phase contrast and dark field microscope into my practice when I was taken to another one of these special healing prayer group evenings. Diane was thirty-seven years old, the mother of seven children, and had been diagnosed with breast cancer. She had already had a round of radiation and chemotherapy. Her status was critical and her situation somewhat desperate. We circled around her, about thirty of us, in the small chapel of a convent, laying on hands and asking for her recovery.

Before the session started, I had proceeded to take a drop of blood from her, for future observation of the oxidative mechanisms present. After about fifteen to twenty minutes of intensive prayer, I took another drop of blood. The results were astonishing. The blood taken before was typical of a high degree of degeneration showing a grade 4/4 of oxidative stress. The blood taken after prayer was absolutely restored to a normal state, showing no oxidative stress at all. The question you may all have in mind is this: was she definitively cured?

She was a very sweet lady and everybody was hoping for a miracle for her. I followed up with her two weeks later to look at her blood again. Unfortunately, it was back to its previous degenerative state. This experience, and many others that followed, allowed me to begin to understand why so often spontaneous healings occur momentarily and are not sustained. I think this is because the integration of a new awareness is not supported by a new way of thinking, a change of habits, or a new dietary lifestyle.

Diane had been caught in a reality very hard to escape. Her lack of financial resources and her family responsibilities were overwhelming. Her husband was completely powerless, in spite of his show of affection. As a medical doctor, deep in my heart, I was praying for the day when we could have a real integrative care center where the patient could be fully supported, not only with palliative treatments but also with all of the knowledge that would allow us to understand the root causes of conditions. Then we could offer the resources necessary to make quantum healing happen in its full potential.

At the time of this experience, I didn't have the understanding of quantum physics that could explain how a spiritual event could be reflected in the blood. It was later when I gradually started to put all of the pieces together. Multiple studies have shown that prayer at a distance is effective in the healing of a patient. Plants grow faster if you project positive thoughts onto them. Dr. Goswami, in *The Quantum Doctor,* presented similar studies where meditators isolated in Faraday cages could influence their brain waves.

In my 2009–2011 conference tour Seeing Is Believing, I demonstrated that we could have the same effect on the morphology of the blood with another spiritual approach called the art of giving divine light (a spiritual technique originating from Japan). The experiment showed a very interesting case of a student before and after a significant loss of weight (forty pounds) and a drastic change of diet. Her blood initially showed definitive characteristics of poor nutrition and significant oxidative stress, particularly in the membrane of the red cells. After twenty minutes of being exposed to the art of giving divine light, the blood showed a dramatic change, especially in the live blood sample.

Today, many health practitioners are using live blood analysis to monitor the effects of diet and supplements on morphology of the blood. This has been demonstrated to be very useful as an indicator of a proper dietary regimen and supplements for the client. How I was introduced to the subject was somewhat more dramatic.

One day, a very good friend in his late thirties called me to share bad news. He had just been diagnosed with colon cancer. He was a family man with seven children and, ironically, himself a naturopath practicing colonic therapy. His plan was obviously not to go with standard medicine first for treatment. He wanted to try everything under the sun to solve his problem the natural way. In his quest, he called me a few weeks later with excitement to share his latest discovery: wheat grass and raw live food. At the time, new dietetic information for cancer was of great interest to me. I immediately began investigating the subject further and didn't lose any time in registering myself for two weeks at the Hippocrates Health Institute in Florida to study. Today, this institute is world-renowned and is still under the direction of Dr. Brian Clement and Dr. Anna Maria Gahns-Clement. There is now profuse literature online about this particular diet created by Ann Wigmore, a pioneer in this field who cured herself of her own breast cancer.

This was very revealing when I experienced the energizing effect of a 100 percent raw-food diet complemented with wheat grass and at the same time witnessed people coming from all over the world trying to improve their cancer situation. A live blood analysis was performed before and after two weeks of a raw diet with wheat grass. Not only did I feel reenergized, but the visual analysis of a small drop of blood demonstrated an incredible improvement. I also noticed that most of the participants were more highly motivated to adhere to their change of nutritional habits when they had a visual, such as the live blood analysis, compared to that of a standard analysis. The compliance to the diet by patients with hypercholesterolemia or type II diabetes, for example, was very low after referring them to a dietician, generally only one to two months, compared to a year of continuing on the diet with review of their live blood analysis.

After a few months passed, my friend, having exhausted everything he could do, decided to visit me. I had already equipped my clinic with a high-phase contrast and dark field microscope. When I saw him, I was shocked. He looked so pale and had obviously lost weight. I performed a live blood analysis and saw that his blood was exhibiting high oxidative stress with anemia and secondarily the colonic cancer, which we already knew. This visual analysis helped me to convince him that it was time to go for surgery and remove the tumor. He willingly let go of his attachment to solve the problem totally naturally and went for surgery in the next few days. Without any further medical treatments, he was completely cured. Today, he is a happy grandpa with many grandchildren.

I see those days as the beginning of integrative medicine, when I was discovering that both natural and standard medicine can work together hand in hand. Alternative approaches could, in many cases, reduce the side effects of an aggressive chemotherapy or radiation treatment.

Chronic Fatigue Syndrome

Originally, I was using live and dry blood analysis to monitor the bioterrain with an approach called the five pillars (discussed in chapter 6). This additional information, when added to the regular diagnostic analysis, provided me with clues that helped thousands of patients.

Chronic fatigue syndrome became almost a specialty. The intent was not to diagnose but to monitor specific parameters that would help me follow the evolution of the client regarding changes in nutritional habits or supplementation. Trained as a medical doctor, I was accustomed to following up with standard medical analysis, so in the beginning I felt very uncomfortable with natural approaches, whereas many other practitioners were proceeding without any assessment.

The point I'm making here is that without any doubt, the blood can reflect the activity going on in the physical body. Live blood analysis has been criticized and questioned in many ways, but with the proper knowledge and professionalism, it can be a significant complementary tool for a creative integrative medical doctor.

Vital Body

To take it one step further, can vital body approaches to healing such as acupuncture, homeopathy, or others including quantum biofeedback, have an effect on blood morphology? By a vital body approach, I mean energetic modalities that have the possibility of influencing nonlocal subtle anatomies like meridians or chakras (as described by Dr. Goswami). My first choice of assessment tools for the vital body had been Kirlian photography and an electro-analysis device, such as Vega testing. But I later discovered that the blood could also be sensitive to energetic therapies.

I soon discovered that German doctors have been open to these ideas for quite a while. Excited by my urge to know more about energetic medicine, I decided to travel to Germany to participate in a world convention on alternative medicine hosted in Baden-Baden. I was exposed firsthand to the work of Peter Mendel in Kirlian photography and other technologies. His work and that of others on this subject seemed most serious about having color pictures of the chakras. There was a science behind it and a refinement needed to interpret these pictures, which revealed a visual map of activity in the meridians and toxicity of the vital body.

The information aspect of stimulated electro-photonic emissions around the human body and other objects has been studied for several decades. Subsequent to the original work of Semion Kirlian, Konstantin Korotkov, a physicist from St. Petersburg Tech University in Russia, developed a new generation of equipment called solid-state computerized gas discharge visualization (GDV). It appears that Kirlian images in some way have provided for alternative medicine doctors what radiology provides to medical doctors. I couldn't resist adding this tool to my practice, in conjunction with a Vega device, which helped me to monitor thousands of patients on homeopathic or acupuncture treatments. With these tools, I could easily recognize energetic imbalances and degree of toxicity in my patients and track how they improved with energetic treatment modalities. This information provided the feedback I needed to successfully integrate alternative modalities with conventional medical treatments.

One day, a lady in her late forties walked into my office. She was desperate. She had already consulted her family doctor many times for an uncomfortable and unusual burning sensation on her scalp. In desperation for a cause, the family doctor had referred her to a dermatologist who, not knowing what to do to, referred her on to a psychiatrist. The psychiatrist prescribed an anxiolytic (antianxiety drug) and recommended a vacation to Florida. Living in Québec, this is the first destination you think of to get away and relax. She was insulted that she wasn't taken seriously. What more could I do?

First, listen with respect. Then, as with many other patients who came to consult with me for problems that regular medicine couldn't solve, look at the situation from another angle: the bio-energetic terrain. In her case, a live blood analysis and Kirlian photography revealed a high degree of toxicity and degenerative forms in her blood. After a few weeks of a proper diet and homeopathy, these parameters were reversed and her condition completely was restored.

I am completely aware that this story is not supported by the kind of scientific research that will turn the skepticism of a scientific community around. But think about how this situation and many similar ones have generated pain, suffering, and frustration, without even considering the energy and money lost for the patients and society. In contrast, what I recommended to this client was less costly and solved a problem that would likely have resulted in interminable care. The majority of the time, this type of client ends up on antidepressants, which just makes them more miserable. I could recount hundreds of stories like this one, with unusual symptoms that leave the medical doctors completely perplexed and that can't be solved easily unless looked at from another perspective.

I believe that in the future, these tools that reveal the body's subtle energy anatomy will be part of the conventional investigation, taking into account what is most important for a comprehensive holistic understanding of the patient. Fortunately, quantum physics provides a premise of understanding that will open the door to the integration of both new and ancient models of healing.

Chapter 6
A New Perspective on Patient Evaluation

One of the most interesting things I learned when I was at medical school was the evaluation of a patient. I soon realized that the difference between a very skilled clinician and an ordinary one was the effectiveness of their clinical evaluation. The questionnaire, a collection of symptoms and clinical signs, could quickly reveal the majority of issues facing the patient, even before lab tests were requested. I was fascinated by how the observation of a patient could reveal so much information. With the primary information gathered, the selection of lab tests and further exams could be more efficient. But never forget that, traditionally, the main goal is to find out what's wrong with the patient. In other words, medical doctors are trained to find the disease, and the better you are at that, the better doctor you are considered to be.

I remember one day early on in my own practice. A very well-known client was living in the town where I was doing my first consultations as a young medical doctor just out of university. When you are starting a medical practice in the country, you have to in some way prove yourself. I was certainly not the first person you would consult for a major health issue, but this notable client had already consulted everybody else in the area and had even gone to the emergency room one weekend in desperation before he knocked on my door. Having just graduated as a medical doctor, I had the advantage of having in mind more possibilities for diagnostics and, unfortunately for him, I diagnosed lymphoma. This diagnosis established my reputation from the beginning, and I became the hero of this little town. From that day forward, everybody consulted me, knowing that if they had something serious, I would find it. I was a good doctor. I still believe that this is how a good conventional doctor should be—one who can identify the problems.

Many years later, when I began to study acupuncture, homeopathy, and naturopathy, I discovered that those disciplines provided more angles from which I could look at my clients. I initially thought that these complementary medicines should all have something in common, but I soon realized that they were each providing different frames of reference for analysis, each with their own language and parameters with which to look at a client. I realized that all systems of healing were revealing different layers of information regarding a more complex reality.

Perhaps the most important realization I had through applying this expanded integrative approach is that patient evaluation is not just about finding the problem or disease. Additional information about their bioterrain (biophysical, emotional, mental, and spiritual terrain) can be obtained and, when all areas are addressed, lead to restoring them to optimum health. This is what creative integrative medicine is about—seeing the unseen or the immaterial aspects of the individual in order to grasp a different quality of information that can be categorized as the vital, mental, or supramental levels of a subtle energy anatomy. It is about understanding the individual globally, looking at parameters that not only guide a doctor to an understanding of what is going wrong but also discovering which elements need to be rebalanced so that the full potential of the client can be restored.

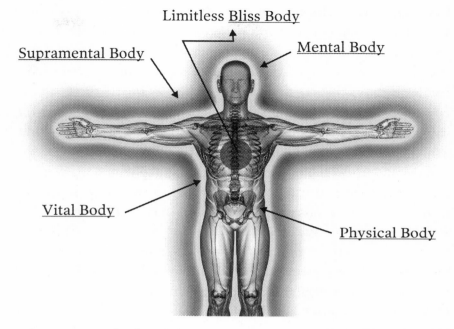

Limitless <u>Bliss Body</u>

<u>Supramental Body</u>

<u>Mental Body</u>

<u>Vital Body</u>

<u>Physical Body</u>

Figure 6.1: Levels of a subtle energy anatomy (Quantum Doctor Course)

Developing a New Model of Observation

In their process of evaluation, the creative integrative doctor should look at an individual from a different perspective than a traditional Western doctor does, meaning considering more health parameters that will lead the client toward full potential. They will ask questions, such as the following:

- What will be the parameters of reference, not only to evaluate what's going on with my patient but also to assess their improvement?

- How long should a client be on a particular diet? Are the homeopathic products used working?

- Is the acupuncture treatment making a difference in the energy field of the client?

Coming from a conventional scientific background (even though I felt this perspective was incomplete), I still believed we should have a systematic way by which to evaluate a client and establish a treatment plan. That is why I looked into the field of complementary medicine to see if there were supplementary evaluation tools that I could use. This led me to travel throughout the world searching for such instruments. Every year Baden-Baden, Germany, hosted a world convention that ultimately introduced me to Volt and Vega electrodermal devices, Kirlian photography, thermography, and many other types of technologies from MORA therapy to laser therapy, just to mention a few. I was fascinated. Later on in America, I was introduced to phase contrast and dark field microscopy or computerized analysis—energetic computers. Each of these new assessment tools provided me with information that didn't have any correlation with the conventional model of medicine. For that reason, though useful, they weren't recognized as being scientific.

Another major step in developing this new model of observation was to establish a methodology for collecting and organizing the diverse qualities of these parameters in reference to different levels of information. If we are looking in terms of what has to be done to bring the client to their full potential, this obviously creates a different perspective. In defining this new and more profound perspective, the limited scope of a materialistic approach based solely on anatomy, chemistry, and biology was insufficient. The frames of reference for observation I chose were from systems of healing more ancient than conventional Western medicine itself. I found a solid basis in establishing this model by referring to the ideas incorporated in ancient systems of healing, such as Taoist medicine and acupuncture, Ayurvedic medicine, homeopathy, and naturopathy. It took me many more years to find the common ground for all modalities of medicine—through the depths of reality as revealed by quantum physics.

Integrating Models from Ancient Systems of Healing

Naturopathy

In naturopathy, I applied the system of the five pillars of health. (See figure 6.2 below.) This system has been used by naturopaths for many years in the assessment of a patient's physical level of health. Instead of only looking at the disease, the clinician collects all relevant information related to a patient's assimilation, detoxification, immunity, oxidation, and regeneration. These parameters can be collected either through dark field-phase contrast microscopy or through other bioterrain laboratory analyses.

Five Pillars of Health

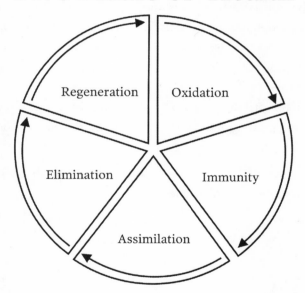

Figure 6.2: Five Pillars of Health (Five Pillars of Health Course)

In the naturopathic approach, these pillars of health guide the health-care practitioner in making the proper choice of supplements or nutrients that will best help their patient. These basic questions— how the client assimilates or detoxifies—are already established in the culture of the naturopathic practitioner, but many ignore these in their choice of therapies. So many times I have seen these practitioners suggesting products systematically, without doing a proper evaluation. Similar questions must also be asked about immunity, oxidation, and regeneration in order to determine a prioritized treatment approach that will lead toward full restoration of health.

Ignoring these basic questions will have as a consequence the client quitting an overwhelming therapy where the long-term cost of therapy is unsustainable. One of the principles of the Hippocratic Oath is "Do no harm." Most of the time, naturopathic practitioners take for granted that natural products have no side effects, which is completely erroneous. Not only is this a blind approach, but overwhelming the client is one of the major reasons for noncompliance and can also have negative consequences. In homeopathy, the healing crisis is a very common consequence of an aggressive therapy. In naturopathy, too many supplements can overload the client in their ability to detoxify or can create undesirable side effects.

One of the basic principles that should be taught in any curriculum of natural and integrative medicine is to try to find the optimal prescription for a client, which is

1. the minimal amount of a product or therapy that will produce the maximum effect; and

2. an approach based on problems and priorities that have been established in a previous evaluation.

We must keep in mind that everything can't be done at once. This principle is obvious, but it is not respected by most natural practitioners. In their anxiety to get results faster, they literally swamp their client with products or therapies.

Conventional medicine is often criticized by the tenants of natural medicine as being focused on symptoms and too dependent on pharmaceuticals. But surprisingly, most of the time, the same pattern of therapeutic behavior is simply transposed into the natural medicine practice, without even preceding it with any kind of evaluation.

By changing only one component of the equation to using natural products instead of a pharmaceutical compound, some practitioners assume that everything is fine and there is no need for proper education and training. Miraculous products and miraculous cures are proposed without any preevaluation or differentiation for the clientele. Some products or cures are advertised as a fit for all.

As long as the basic practices of natural medicine or any other type of energetic medicine are not based first on a proper scientific foundation and on a more step-by-step method of evaluation, natural and complementary medicines won't be respected within the realm of modern medicine. Again, this is what creative integrative medicine is about—providing the premises of scientific models of observation and evaluation to guide doctors from many avenues or disciplines toward an understanding of the globalism of the client. This, in turn, will enable them to lead their client toward his or her full potential.

I found the five pillars approach very useful in organizing the patient's information in my own practice, especially when using dark field microscopy blood analysis and the basic naturopathy questionnaire. This was also the concept used in a computer software program that I designed to organize the results for blood analysis microscopy, using high-phase contrast and dark field analysis. In Montreal, where I had established a research institute, we collected data using phase contrast and dark field blood microscopy. Four microscopists used the five pillars model to standardize an evaluation methodology (which was typically qualitative and based on the morphology of the blood) into a more quantitative one. After a blood analysis report, we were able to determine how the five pillars were graded from I to V, which provided us with a more accurate view of the bioterrain of the client.

This proved to be very useful when doing a client consult for chronic diseases or cancer. Unfortunately, most patients in this situation feel they are confronted with the choice of either a medical or a natural approach to treatment. This is sad, since these two approaches can be integrated together very effectively. As a medical doctor also knowledgeable in other complementary medicines, my first responsibility before making any choices was to look first at the whole picture. Yes, we should have a medical diagnosis, but we should also have a deeper view of what I call the bioterrain—the physical, vital, mental (including emotional), supramental, and spiritual aspects of a client.

The five pillars approach, in particular, informed me which resources of this patient were challenged by the major stress of a chronic disease or cancer. After the cancer was medically evaluated and graded, the same assessment could be addressed differently in terms of the biophysical terrain. I found many times, for example, that the degree of toxicity determined by the lifestyle and long-term bad habits of patients would influence how they responded to alternative therapies.

Regarding their immunity, the load of pathogens was a major issue. A lot of research has been done and literature published on the yeast syndrome and parasites, but most of the time, the medical mainstream doesn't even acknowledge it.

Yet another major concern to address is the level of oxidation—in other terms, how my patient is dealing with free radicals. Cancer creates a highly oxidative situation in the body, and I found that some patients would cope better than others with the disease. The level of oxidation is quite a reliable gauge of how fast the cancer is evolving and how much more aggressive we should be with complementary approaches.

And what about the pillar of assimilation, which is also compromised and makes oral products useless if they can't be assimilated?

In chapter 2, I described aspects of spontaneous healing that also apply to the pillar of regeneration, a reality completely unacknowledged in the medical world but probably more important than the future of genetic medicine.

Many times, I found patients unrealistically refusing a conventional medical approach to cancer, thinking that vitamin C alone could be an alternative. In my years of practice, I witnessed clients who used complementary approaches cure their cancer and also those who died. They have taught me many lessons. Even with an open mind, my basic education is still founded in medical and "scientific thought." Even when I heard stories of breast, pancreatic, or other types of cancer being healed, I was sometimes still doubtful. The "heroes of medicine," which is how I recognize them today, that I met either in my own clinics or later on in my various experiences working in other clinics or hospitals, convinced me of the reality of another path of healing. I call these trailblazers "heroes" because they went against all odds and fatalistic diagnoses and searched on their own to find other solutions, using their own resources, despite being judged as crazy, or at least very presumptuous or fantastical. They have taught me that cancer and other chronic diseases must be approached from many levels and require a serious and deep commitment.

The truth about these diseases is that they are multifactorial and must be addressed on all levels. In conventional medicine, we like to find one bad guy and go after it with the strongest drugs. In the context of holistic medicine, this is a different and problematic issue with multiple components and should be addressed globally. Attention should not be focused only on the physical or nutritional but also on the vital, emotional, mental, and sometimes spiritual components. Many researchers have confirmed the emotional component of cancer.

My point here is that a comprehensive holistic evaluation is required from the start. In the case of a cancer, for example, there is no doubt that the evaluation must be graded medically. However, a bioterrain (physical, vital, mental …) analysis also must be done in order to determine more accurately not only what the resources of the patient are but how many factors are involved and what work must be done to reverse the imbalance and create an environment for optimal healing and regeneration. It is crucial to understand that our intention here is directed toward an understanding of what the multilevel factors are (physical, emotional, mental, spiritual ...) and engage the client in a positive mode of healing. The reality of this approach is that it will require active involvement by the client, where they will have to change habits, lifestyle, and ways of thinking and do emotional and spiritual work. There is no magic pill here. The magic is found in quantum creativity, a subject that we addressed in chapter 2.

This is why this first step of a detailed patient evaluation is so important— to help guide the patient in making a realistic choice of integrative therapies. An integrative approach should never discourage the client from conventional medical therapy but should instead integrate conventional medical therapy as part of a more global treatment plan. Creative integrative medicine will one day be part of the health care of the future and will provide patients with many more alternatives, making all forms of therapies more efficient.

Taoist Medicine and Acupuncture

Taoist medicine and the Five Elements was another natural healing system I used as a frame of reference for observation. I found it very useful to refer to this model to track the movement of energy in the vital body along the meridians, their associated organs, and related emotions. Not only has this model been used for centuries, but I think it also provides precious information on emotions that could be used to solve the mind-body conflict.

In Taoist medicine, meridians are related to organs and also have different types of personalities. I find Taoist and acupuncture medicine fascinating in how it reveals in a more accurate fashion how diseases originate, but even more so, how to prevent them.

Morphogenetic fields and their relationships through the five elements have been refined by Taoist medicine for centuries.

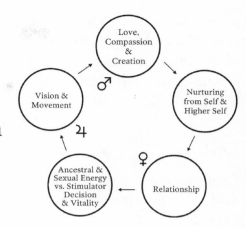

Figure 6.3: Morphogenetic fields and their relationships through the Five Elements (Quantum Taoist Medicine and Acupuncture Course)

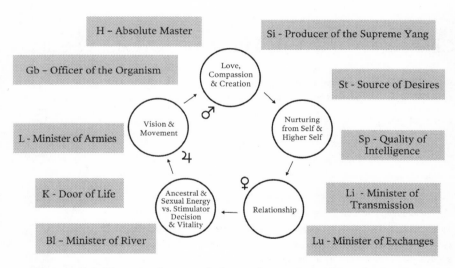

Figure 6.4: The meridians and their relationships through the Five Elements (Quantum Taoist Medicine and Acupuncture Course)

Ancient acupuncturists already knew that by observing the pulses, you could determine the status of meridians and their related organs, and by puncturing specific points, restore balance and prevent the manifestation of disease. Today's practitioners of energetic medicine in Europe (more specifically in Germany) now have a visual representation of the meridians through Kirlian photography. I used and became familiar with this medium when practicing medicine in Canada. This was for me an important tool for evaluation, not only to have a visual representation of the meridian system but also to show the movement of energy in the vital body.

Chakras

Complementary to the Taoist acupuncture model, I incorporated the model of chakras described in Ayurvedic medicine and as mentioned by Dr. Goswami. This adds further refinement to the model of emotions revealed by the previous system. "Feelings are the experience of the chakra's vital energy, the movements of your morphogenetic fields," says Dr. Goswami in *The Quantum Doctor* (2004, 142).

Chakras & Vital Body Functions, Organs, & Glands

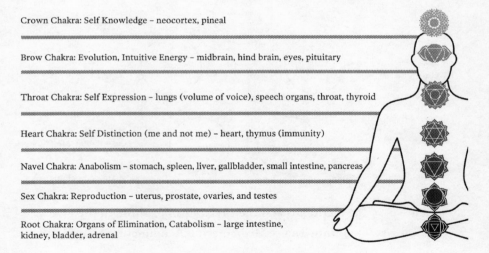

Crown Chakra: Self Knowledge – neocortex, pineal

Brow Chakra: Evolution, Intuitive Energy – midbrain, hind brain, eyes, pituitary

Throat Chakra: Self Expression – lungs (volume of voice), speech organs, throat, thyroid

Heart Chakra: Self Distinction (me and not me) – heart, thymus (immunity)

Navel Chakra: Anabolism – stomach, spleen, liver, gallbladder, small intestine, pancreas

Sex Chakra: Reproduction – uterus, prostate, ovaries, and testes

Root Chakra: Organs of Elimination, Catabolism – large intestine, kidney, bladder, adrenal

Figure 6.5: Chakras and vital body functions, organs and glands (Quantum Doctor Course)

Organs, Glands, Chakras, Dominant Feelings

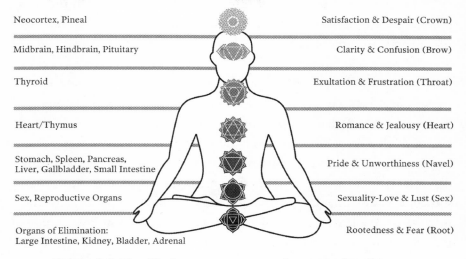

Neocortex, Pineal

Midbrain, Hindbrain, Pituitary

Thyroid

Heart/Thymus

Stomach, Spleen, Pancreas,
Liver, Gallbladder, Small Intestine

Sex, Reproductive Organs

Organs of Elimination:
Large Intestine, Kidney, Bladder, Adrenal

Satisfaction & Despair (Crown)

Clarity & Confusion (Brow)

Exultation & Frustration (Throat)

Romance & Jealousy (Heart)

Pride & Unworthiness (Navel)

Sexuality-Love & Lust (Sex)

Rootedness & Fear (Root)

Figure 6.6: The Chakra energy system showing related organs, glands and dominant feelings (Quantum Doctor Course)

But still, I feel that these concepts exposing an energetic reality, as defined through Taoist medicine, acupuncture, and Ayurvedic traditions, must be supported by a more scientific foundation. Research based on new premises of quantum physics and more sophisticated tools of investigation will allow us to explore these concepts in more depth in the future.

Moving a Patient toward Positive Health

As we previously mentioned, how we perceive things matters in quantum physics, and it matters even more in the evaluation process. A fundamental difference between a conventional evaluation and the creative integrative evaluation is the qualitative information provided by the additional parameters. The perspective differs in that in conventional medicine the intent is to find the diagnosis: What's wrong here? What is the patho-physiologic process that is affecting the individual here? In the new integrative model, the information obtained is not only an attempt to understand what's going on, but in more global terms, it includes many layers of information (physical, vital, mental, supramental, and spiritual) that can be used to provide guidance as to what must be improved or reinforced for the client to reach their full potential.

But how do you define full potential? Dr. Deepak Chopra wrote about perfect health, a concept that was translated by Dr. Goswami into positive health. What I found interesting about this idea of positive health is that it is not just about performance but also more about integration. This correlation between emotions and meridians, already discussed in Taoist and acupuncture medicine, has more depth than someone could imagine by relating simple emotions to organs and meridians. People who are familiar with the concepts know, for example, that the heart is associated with love and hate and the kidneys with courage and fear.

Dr. Amit Goswami, in his book *The Quantum Doctor* (2004), was a pioneer in correlating the systems of meridians to the vital body as a nonlocal reality, based on the work of Rupert Sheldrake and his research on the morphogenetic field. The contribution of Dr. Goswami to creative integrative medicine, applying the principles of quantum physics, such as nonlocality, tangled hierarchy, and a discontinuous leap in consciousness, is tremendous for modern medicine. I believe that in a few years, these notions will be seen as the fundamental template for the scientific basis for creative integrative medicine and will be taught at medical schools.

The vital body, as described by Dr. Goswami, provides the foundation for the first layer of information concerning the concept of vital energy that is described by the ancient healing systems of acupuncture, Ayurvedic medicine, naturopathy, and homeopathy. The five pillars were designed more for the physical level but can now be organized into more subtle information regarding the vital body as well.

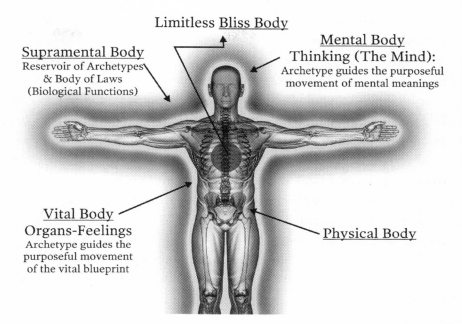

Limitless Bliss Body

Supramental Body
Reservoir of Archetypes
& Body of Laws
(Biological Functions)

Mental Body
Thinking (The Mind):
Archetype guides the purposeful
movement of mental meanings

Vital Body
Organs-Feelings
Archetype guides the
purposeful movement
of the vital blueprint

Physical Body

Figure 6.7: Levels of a subtle energy body (Quantum Doctor Course)

Another level of information is the mental body, a reservoir of mental meanings. Today, I would compare this compartment to what we call mind-body medicine and psychosomatic medicine. The connection with the mind can't be denied any longer, although the conventional model of medicine is stuck with a dualistic approach to mind and body. The concept of Dr. Goswami's "consciousness as the ground of all being" offers the point of view that mind and brain are both possibilities of consciousness. This creates a new understanding of a comprehensive approach in looking at how the mind interacts with the body. This will also add to the evaluation process new avenues with which to explore the common reality in which clients facing degenerative, psychosomatic diseases and cancers are trapped.

The concept of positive health brings us to another layer of information, which is the supramental level. As defined by Dr. Goswami, the supramental is the reservoir of archetypes and body of laws (or biological functions). If the vital body contains the blueprint of the organs, or what

Sheldrake describes as the morphologic fields, where does the innate intelligence that provides this information reside? The answer is in the supramental, a layer of information without representation, reflecting our inner intuition—something already known by the Taoist masters. Transpersonal psychology, humanistic philosophy, and many others like Carl Gustav Jung have described universal qualities that can be recognized when an individual becomes more mature or whole. This is what positive health is about—looking at the individual not only through a range of various emotions, but also looking at how these emotions and feelings have evolved from a personal ego level to a more universal one. Health is not only physical but also vital, emotional, mental, and spiritual.

Taoist masters described what we call the "Rainbow Body," a subtle energetic body, a

> complex of meridians, avenues of waves, colored by the density of their vibration, that are fast or slow, strong or weak, according to the individual mind's reaction to the personal and social events of life—whether joyful or sad. One day every meridian of the Rainbow Body will be in perfect harmony ...

where qualities of the soul will have evolved from an ego mode, through a self mode, to a more universal value. "Then the physical body will never fall ill and the blood will sing in all the vessels of the body" (de Surany, le Corps d'Arc en Ciel (The Rainbow Body) 1996).

We went into more detail in chapter 2 about the concept of personal growth and quantum leaps, which are key to quantum creativity and spontaneous healing. At this time, I would like to stress that the evaluation process involves more than finding the problem or disease. There is a more profound definition of health that encompasses the notion of absence of pain and a greater sense of well-being and happiness that can be seen in the energetic apparatus of the client. As body language reveals the individual, there is also an energetic signature that will guide the clinician through different layers of information.

Today, when the client or patient walks in the office of a doctor, they should be aware that the doctor is looking to find out what is wrong with him or her. Without this comprehensive view of subtle energy anatomy and a process of evaluation that is looking not only at deadly parameters but more at life parameters, the patient/client is caught in a fatalistic approach where there are no possibilities for regeneration, balancing, restoration, or personal growth toward a greater experience of reality. In the future, when he or she will go to see a creative integrative doctor, this doctor should not only be able to see a deeper perspective but also be able to tap into layers of information that have the possibility of helping restore their full potential.

Bio-Vital-Mental-Supramental-Bliss Terrain

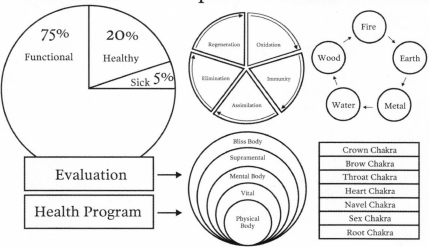

Figure 6.8: Bio-Vital-Mental-Supramental-Bliss Terrain (Five Pillars of Health Course)

In conclusion, the ancient models of healing or naturopathy described throughout the book can come together on a foundation offered by the model of quantum physics, as described by Dr. Goswami. Figure 6.8

above can help the clinician to organize information more coherently in accordance with the concepts taught at the Quantum University. These frames of reference provide the clinician with a map to track the movement of the subtle energy in a client in relation to their feelings, emotions, meridians, chakras, and organs and to have a broader perspective of their physical-emotional-mental-spiritual bioterrain. How can we ignore centuries of knowledge of models of healing that have already explored the mind and body connection? Quantum physics bridges the ancient and the modern in many ways, providing a more accurate language and a reasonable scientific ground to make this knowledge available to a modern creative integrative medicine.

Chapter 7
Creating a New Paradigm for Medical Education

Why We Need a New Paradigm for Medical Education

At present, as I am writing these lines, there is a furious debate in America about health care. Without going into the politics of it, I wonder whether we are really paying attention to the right questions. During my career, I have been exposed to two different models of medicine: a socialized system in Canada and a private insurance-based system in America. The real problem, no matter what your strategy is for paying your medical bills, is that neither system will be able to afford the rising costs of conventional medicine. Is it not clear that conventional medicine, with too few means of treatment—pharmaceuticals, surgery, and now genetics—is out of reach of our budgets?

The foreword of this book states, "Nobody knows the price we are paying for an incomplete model of medical education." Have we for one moment in this crucial debate heard about or questioned what foundation our medical education is based upon? How health-care practitioners are trained and educated? Is there another way to look at the reality of healing? Is there another way of restoring health and providing a cure?

When I was studying in medical school, the first three years were spent learning sciences, such as human anatomy and physiology, chemistry, microbiology, biochemistry, genetics, immunology, neurology, and hematology. Later on, I was taught about diseases related to the body's pulmonary, cardiovascular, gastrointestinal, genitourinary, endocrine, reproductive, and other systems. With your brain full of all this information, you walk through the corridors of a hospital in white coats with stethoscopes around your necks for another three years, trying to make sense of how to heal people. And don't forget, two or three nights a week you must be on duty at a hospital, meaning that many times you could be awake and working for thirty-six hours in a row. I am not enthusiastic about this tradition of education, but we have to recognize the merits of those that have walked these initiatory paths.

But what is deceiving here is that the medical system is missing a complete understanding of the mechanics of healing. Missing from the picture is the reality of the *unseen,* which, according to quantum physics, includes more than 99 percent of what we have consciously perceived or acknowledged to date. The remainder (less than 1 percent) is matter and represents the layer of information that medical science deals with today.

This is the main message of this book—to introduce for the next generation of physicians a new model of education based on the premise of looking at reality from the point of view of quantum physics, which opens up infinite possibilities for healing. The idea is not to erase what we have acquired until now through science and technology. Rather it is to integrate this knowledge into a broader model of understanding and to incorporate modalities of healing that require an acknowledgment of subtle energies that exist and cause effects beyond what the linear model of biology, chemistry, and conventional physics shows us.

This was my objective in creating Quantum University—to add the missing pieces of the puzzle, which will allow medicine to deal with 100 percent of the reality for a person's healing. A pretentious task?

The Founding of International Quantum University for Integrative Medicine (IQUIM)

As I explained in the introduction, the death of my brother in my teenage years was the primary catalyst for me to engage on the path to becoming a medical doctor. Through reading the subsequent chapters, you have probably noticed that this first initiative took many turns after I began my journey. Going through a conventional medical system of education didn't satisfy my burning desire for healing or provide me with an in-depth understanding of the real art of medicine.

While on this journey, I realized that it was imperative that a quantum integrative model of healing should be embedded in the curriculum of a university. This is the typical way that a society embraces new paradigm shifts. But where do you start? I had no idea how the universe would play out the realization of how this would happen. During the years that Quantum University took form, I faced many challenges. I thought that readers would be interested to know what the major challenges encountered were.

When I first came to America, I faced many handicaps. My English was not fluent and I was literally unknown. Like many others who have come to America with a dream, I had to start at "ground zero." A few years ago, when I received my US citizenship and looked back over my twelve years in America, I could acknowledge that this land provides a privileged environment, one which has allowed my original desire to heal to come to maturity. Similar to others who have come here, I too can say that America is the land of the impossible dream, even if I feel that this is just the first bloom's bud.

In the beginning, I gave various lectures and workshops with a French accent that was not always favorable. One day when I was living in San Diego, another synchronistic event occurred. A friend invited me to Encinitas to visit the California Institute for Human Science (CIHS). There I was introduced to the director of research. I presented myself in quite a bad French-English accent. Surprisingly, he answered me back in French. Dr. Gaetan Chevalier, a PhD and physicist originally from Montreal, was already pursuing his career in the United States. Dr. Chevalier went on to play a key role in the beginning and evolution of Quantum University.

At that time, I was just starting to lecture on a very popular subject known as quantum biofeedback. Many users of a new computerized technology associated with biofeedback were in need of additional training and education. More importantly, they didn't have any professional status or credentials. With the support of Dr. Chevalier, I initiated a training program based on the fundamentals of biofeedback, mixed with elements of quantum medicine. The original training course met the requirements of the Neurotherapy and Biofeedback Certification Board (NBCB). It enabled practitioners in the field of biofeedback to become board certified, with specific qualifications for using biofeedback for stress reduction as their scope of practice.

This was the onset of a series of lectures I gave that exposed me to thousands of natural medicine practitioners in major cities across the United States and Canada. As I traveled, I recognized that there was a need for a more comprehensive education for these dedicated students. In fact, most of them were looking for a practice of natural medicine that would encompass the scope of a biofeedback practitioner.

Which brings me to the subject of "professional status and credentials" in the field of natural medicine. This issue was prevalent in Canada as well as in the United States. Too often, practitioners of natural medicine, or in this case a biofeedback technology, didn't have proper training or sufficient education. While conventional medicine is generally criticized by the mainstream of natural medicine practitioners, one has to agree that the majority of licensed medical professionals have gone through a well-defined system of education and training. I am quite knowledgeable about this subject, since I myself participated in this extensive training to become a medical doctor.

Earlier on in Canada, as well as in America, I recognized the lack of formal systemized education in the fields of natural medicine or complementary and alternative medicine. What I had noticed was what I call the "workshop syndrome." In other words, many people gather as many weekend workshop certificates as they can in an attempt to jump into a natural medicine or biofeedback practice, thinking they're gaining the competence and knowledge required to deal with complex health-care issues.

For this reason, I began to focus my efforts on building a curriculum of information that was first recognized as a certification program in biofeedback, then in traditional naturopathy. This explains why the International Quantum University for Integrative Medicine (IQUIM) was originally known as International Quantum Biofeedback Natural Medicine (IQBNM). It had evolved from a school offering a certification program to a university now offering bachelor's, master's, and PhD level degree programs in both natural and integrative medicine.

Addressing Student Challenges

The good news was that with the new status of IQUIM's degree programs, we could welcome hundreds of these students, often self-educated through years of seminars and weekend workshops, and provide them with a form of recognition for all of their efforts dedicated to learning natural medicine. As the years passed, this idea of expanding the scope of practice of biofeedback practitioners appeared to be rewarding to those who chose this path, which leads to the next story.

Teresa's Story

One day when I was in Canada for a conference, I met Teresa. She was a biofeedback practitioner offering her services from a small office in her backyard. What was special about her? I recognized at first sight that she was a gifted healer having a hard time supporting her five children with her main source of income. Like many others who consider going into the field of healing and respond to their genuine desire to heal others, she faced the challenges of financing and time availability. As the only provider for her five children, life didn't give her the opportunity to go to medical school, and she obviously didn't have the finances to be able to invest in her education. She also had to face the hard reality of when she would have time to study, when she already had her hands full with work and her family.

I had already reflected on these types of difficult situations before initiating the university and had come to the conclusion that in society, even when there is an urgent need for health-care practitioners, the process to become one of them is not easy and often disqualifies many of its best potential candidates. Medical doctors are selected for medical school based on their GPA, which usually reveals that the student has ability in mathematics and physics. Many people recognize today that gifted healers are not necessarily the ones that perform the best at school in those subjects. To counteract this issue when founding the university, I intentionally chose some of the core mission statements to be the following mission and belief statements:

- We believe that the right to heal belongs to everyone who sincerely manifests and desires it.
- We believe that everyone should be educated on how to heal themselves and others. (IQUIM, Mission and Belief Statements)

Since the university was able to acknowledge Teresa's previous education and training, she was able to qualify for admission to the program. But this still did not solve her financial situation or time-availability challenges.

Another one of my personal beliefs is that if you have a real desire to help others (heal others) and this is your mission, then the universe will provide you in time with what is needed to make this happen. What was required of her was a little leap of faith, the same trust that she would later on teach her clients—that something greater is in control here and that the universe is playing in their favor for healing.

Based on this principle, Quantum University began offering an in-house financing program with no interest and no credit check to allow students, with a minimal payment every month, to afford their education. As this policy was implemented, we realized that with the extra credentials and knowledge they were acquiring, the students were able to generate, almost from the start, more income than needed to generously cover the monthly tuition fee.

With additional foresight, we decided to associate the degree programs with different levels of certification in specific disciplines, so that even if students had not completed the full program, they could already practice a few alternative modalities. This created a tremendous advantage in that most of our students have already paid off all of their tuition by the time they complete their degree and don't have to carry the burden of a student loan.

Now what about the availability factor? One objection that we often hear from potential students is "When will I have the time to study?" I went through the same challenge myself. When practicing medicine in Canada, I was busy with hundreds of patients a week and was starting a family with two children. It was at that time that I acquired my complementary alternative medical studies, as outlined in the introduction. My strategy was simple: do a little every day. I would wake up one hour before everybody else in the morning, and as I was studying, I would use a tape recorder to record the most difficult material and replay it during the day for memorization. With this strategy, I acquired multiple additional diplomas and certifications. Later on, I expanded on this idea with my son, Alexi, to use a more advanced platform for education, the iPad, to allow Quantum University students to do the same—to have a more effective tool for time management.

The story of Teresa did have a happy ending. She was able to sign up for her program and eventually became a doctor of natural medicine with a PhD. Her children looked at her as a hero. Very soon afterward, she moved into larger facilities and was able to make a living for her family, while practicing her passion to help others to heal. You can see her story online at http://iquim.org/testimonial-post/terry-conarroe/.

Fostering a Humanitarian Approach: Worldwide Clinics for Humanity

The inspiring story I'm about to tell you shows that the interest in integrative medicine is a worldwide phenomenon. The concept of quantum medicine has been developed over the past fifty years by many thinkers, writers, and doctors inspired by the new paradigm of quantum physics. Over time, more and more students from all parts of the world have inquired about Quantum University and engaged themselves in careers in natural or integrative medicine.

Patricia's Story

Patricia called me one day from Japan. She was on her way to Saudi Arabia and was considering practicing natural medicine. One of her major concerns was how she would be recognized in that part of the world.

Following up on this global need, I contacted Dr. Sheila McKenzie from Canada, who is president of the World Organization of Natural Medicine (WONM). WONM has now become, for students, the major path to recognition for practicing natural medicine in countries that don't have any organizations to provide credentials. WONM has helped a student named Patricia Knox, as well as others on five continents, to become recognized in her legitimate desire to assist others.

During our discussions, Dr. McKenzie also introduced me to her original idea of humanitarian clinics associated with WONM. Medical doctors have Doctors Without Borders, so why should natural medicine not have an equivalent? I was very inspired by the humanitarian work that she was already doing in poor countries and even in Canada. Her Clinics for Humanity in Canada provide services, such as addictions management, nutrition counseling, skills training, and lifestyle management for abused women. The Clinics for Humanity in Haiti provide education for nursing students in community eclectic medicine and village health-care worker training.

My additional question to her was: could the students of Quantum University offer humanitarian services in their own clinics and be recognized by WONM? Her positive response made possible a happy ending for Patricia. Dr. Patricia Knox graduated from Quantum University and became an ambassador of WONM in Saudi Arabia. She initiated a project for the first Clinic for Humanity there, offering an alternative approach to improving outcomes of individuals with autism. You can go online for more details about her story at http://iquim.org/quantum-world-tv/paul-drouin/true-quantum-hero-autism/.

These stories and many others were very enlightening for me and became the subject of many conferences I presented at in America, particularly for the American Naturopathic Medical Association (ANMA).

The "Pay It Forward" Philosophy

Health care is one of the most attractive educational fields leading to prospective employment today. *CNN Money* reports that convincing statistics point in this direction. You may think that the decision to act on this opportunity is an easy one, but not necessarily. One of the problems facing people who choose this path is how to afford the cost of education. The overall debt of students in America is currently one trillion dollars (Herships 2012). Medical students are probably at the top of the list regarding their level of indebtedness (Hopkins 2011). According to the Department of Education's National Center for Education Statistics (NCES), the average cost of a doctoral degree at a public school in 2008 reached $48,400 each year. Private school tuition during the same year rose to $60,000 annually. A typical doctoral program takes five full-time years to complete, bringing the total cost to $242,000 to $300,000 (Institute of Education Sciences 2010).

In seeking further financing solutions for our students, we asked ourselves if there was another way for them to engage in this educational choice without facing the stress of going further into debt. Our answer was yes. *Pay it forward,* which means asking the beneficiary of a good deed to repay it to others instead of to the original benefactor (*Wikipedia*).

It has become obvious to me that the acceptance of natural medicine in our society today is not just a question of regulation or even of scientific data. Too often, natural medicine is presented through a window of financial opportunity based on fact. MSNBC and the Associated Press have reported that thirty-four billion dollars will be spent annually on complementary and alternative medicine (CAM). The perceived association with health products or technologies presented at convention events sometimes creates mistrust in the public. I am not arguing the quality of the good intention of these activities, but they are not helping the cause of a general acceptance of natural or alternative medicines.

Discovering the WONM humanitarian clinics was very refreshing and inspired in me the concept that contributing to society is also an essential part of the equation. With health-care costs becoming more unaffordable, what could be the argument against refusing voluntary services? This is nothing new. In America, medical doctors are already reaching poor communities by offering free medical services. Without any general consensus, many alternative modalities are now present in hospital clinics. Following the same logic, would people refuse help, even if the approach used is natural medicine?

To implement the *"Pay It Forward"* philosophy, Quantum University teamed up with the World Organization of Natural Medicine's Clinics for Humanity and designed a financial aid program that provides students with another way to finance their health-care education: tuition awards. When a student receives a tuition award (which helps to reduce their tuition fees), they then pay it forward by doing voluntary humanitarian services within their community upon graduation (IQUIM, What is a Quantum Hero?).

Pay It Forward tuition awards are, for the students, certainly one of the more creative solutions to the issue of unaffordable health-care education and rising student debt in America. It has become a way in which students can both reduce their tuition costs and contribute to their communities by volunteering their time in the service of humanity. Quantum University, continuously inspired by this idea of humanitarian services, is just in the early stages of a more ambitious project: to generate, with the help of nonprofit organizations, more than ten million dollars' worth of humanitarian services in the years ahead—to offer to communities a significant contribution to health care.

An Advanced Platform for Student Education

As mentioned before, my mission at Quantum University is to educate anyone who is sincere about obtaining an exceptional education in the healing arts, regardless of race, political preference, gender, religion, or financial status. We are looking to attract those who seek the highest level of proficiency as health professionals, so that our students may become the new leaders of the twenty-first century in holistic, alternative, natural, and integrative medicine. In order to increase accessibility to our programs and ensure the success of our students in their education, we have also developed an advanced education platform with tools to assist them in the learning process.

Virtual Learning

As mentioned in Teresa's story earlier, the challenge many students face is this: "How will I find the time to study?" We understand that time is often a major factor for adult students committed to continuing education. They are often juggling family and career commitments, so we decided to give them the technology that will enable them to study and learn from almost anywhere in the world. We decided to offer all courses and materials online through our website or loaded onto an iPad, so that students do not have to invest in a move to the university to be able to take advantage of our programs. With most payment plans, students who enroll in one of our degree programs receive a free iPad loaded with class videos and course documents and other learning assistance programs.

This virtual learning strategy that we have created is designed to save our students both time and money. With no out-of-pocket travel or commute expenses, our online programs can be accessed from a home or office computer or an iPad. This also gives students the flexibility to study at their own pace and view or review course lectures and take exams on their own time, at their convenience, according to their own circumstances and schedule.

"Quantum Superlearning Technology"

After years of advising prospective students, we found that those who had a strong desire to earn a degree yet put off enrolling had one thing in common: they were all afraid that they no longer had the mind power to learn and retain so much new information. In response, we worked with Dr. Porter, the creator of ZenFrames™ and MindFit, to develop a "Quantum Superlearning Technology" to help them overcome these fears and to optimize their ability to focus, learn, and succeed in achieving their academic goals. When developing this technology, we applied the knowledge of the quantum concepts that we teach to enable students to perform at their highest possible level. This system takes into account the knowledge that a whole-brain state and alpha/theta brainwave frequencies create the optimum learning environment and that when learning occurs at the level of quantum consciousness, the information is more easily retained and recalled as needed.

The MindFit specialty glasses are equipped with pulsating light frequencies combined with rhythmic binaural beats, creative visualization/relaxation (CVR), and mind-music to reduce stress and to relax, and to entrain the brain into a state of consciousness that heightens clarity and focus. This helps the student to get motivated, think clearly, stay focused, and easily retain and recall what they have learned, enabling them to review, in this subliminal mode of consciousness, the main points of every lecture. Dr. Porter's recorded voice, in conjunction with the other aspects of the MindFit technology, guides a student through the highlights of each main course subject. These recordings can be loaded onto the student's iPad, along with other bonus relaxing and uplifting meditations and visualizations from Dr. Porter's library.

This technology not only benefits a student's ability to learn but has several added health benefits as well, including increased blood flow to and balancing of the right and left hemispheres of the brain, an increase in serotonin and endorphin levels, a reduced need for sleep, and an increased ability to handle stress (Cady 1990).

This "Quantum Superlearning Technology" is unique to Quantum University and is the first of its kind in the context of an online university. It has realized a lot of success among our students. In many ways, we are trying to not only build a new medical curriculum for integrative medicine based on quantum physics but also to build an education system that incorporates these concepts to enable students to achieve their own maximum potential and enhance their own well-being while going through this learning process.

Building a Curriculum for Creative Integrative Medicine

I feel that the stature of a university is established by the stature of its teachers and its capacity to bring the most exact and updated knowledge in terms of science to society. I believe that an outdated model of science, upon which our current model of health education is based, is in urgent need of being replaced by the new standard of science as defined by quantum physics. It is very clear to me that one individual alone cannot articulate the depth and complexity of this new paradigm. The emergence of creative integrative medicine can't be played as a solo. It must be played as a collective symphony, as an orchestra.

In every century, great minds emerge to redefine a new paradigm within the society. After the popular movie *What the Bleep Do We Know?!* many people were left with a whetted appetite for more of this new knowledge about infinite possibilities. Many of the featured scientists became well-known and added additional books to their credit to deepen the shared knowledge of this new emerging science. Dr. Joe Dispenza's *Breaking the Habit of Being Yourself* (2012) and *You Are the Placebo* (2014), Lynne McTaggart's *The Field* (2008), *The Intention Experiment* (2007), and *The Bond* (2011), Dr. Amit Goswami's *God Is Not Dead* (2008) and *Quantum Creativity* (2014), and Dr. Bruce Lipton's *Biology of Belief* (2005) are just a few. The new stars of a new paradigm in science were born. The one element that had been missing, however, was to bring them all together as a "dream team" of teachers at a university. Due to the law of attraction, many from this group have now joined us at Quantum University.

Bringing together the most important *game changers* in the field of quantum medicine as a dream team of teachers at the university has certainly been a major step in our history, as it allows us the possibility of laying out a new blueprint for a curriculum that will redefine modern medicine as an art of healing.

Teachers to Inspire a New Generation of Health-Care Professionals

Now I would like you to meet the dream team of pioneers and leaders in their fields who are helping to inspire, build, create, and teach a new curriculum for integrative and natural quantum medicine. In conjunction with these teachers, we are building a foundation for education in the areas of quantum physics applied to health and the healing process, biology and evolution, mind-based medicine, energy medicine, auriculotherapy, aromatherapy, natural and integrative medicine, and clinical evaluation and applications.

Quantum Physics Applied to Health and the Healing Process, Biology and Evolution

Dr. Gaetan Chevalier, mentioned earlier, was certainly a source of inspiration from the beginning to initiate what is today Quantum University. I am grateful for what was, at that time, the beginning of a genuine friendship. Early on, through many discussions and connections, he helped me to navigate the process of building a university and was one of the first scientists to implement the principles of quantum physics into a university curriculum. In addition to assisting in the founding of the university, Dr. Chevalier has also developed and teaches our course entitled quantum biology, which introduces the students to concepts of quantum physics and how they impact our views on human biology and evolution.

As I explained in chapter 1, **Dr. Amit Goswami,** through another synchronistic event in the universe, was the first from the select group from *What the Bleep Do We Know?!* to join Quantum University. Dr. Goswami previously served as a professor in the theoretical physics department of the University of Oregon in Eugene from 1968 until his recent retirement. He is the pioneer of "a new paradigm of science" called *science within consciousness.* Dr. Goswami's *Quantum Mechanics* (1991) textbook is used by universities worldwide. He has also written many popular books based on his research on quantum physics and consciousness for nonscientists including *The Physicist's View of Nature,* volumes 1 (2000) and 2 (2001), *The Self-Aware Universe* (1993), *Quantum Creativity* (2014), *The Visionary Window* (2006), *Physics of the Soul* (2001), and *God Is Not Dead* (2008).

Together, we have worked to build the quantum physics foundation for the curriculum of creative integrative medicine at Quantum University. Many of the foundational ideas presented in his books—*The Quantum Doctor* and others—have been expanded on in our courses the quantum doctor, the quantum healer, and the quantum activist.

Lynne McTaggart is an investigative journalist, author, and a sought-after public speaker worldwide who has appeared on several national TV and radio shows including Oprah Winfrey and Deepak Chopra, and in the popular documentaries *What the Bleep Do We Know?!* (Arntz 2004) and *The Living Matrix* (Becker 2009). Her in-depth research into quantum physics, spirituality, and health has culminated in several best-selling books including *The Field* (2008), *The Intention Experiment* (2007), *What Doctors Don't Tell You* (1996), and *The Bond* (2011). She has played an important role in popularizing the concepts of quantum physics. *The Field* is a classic in that field and has been translated in fourteen languages. The field trilogy master class (McTaggart), offered at Quantum University, is a comprehensive course integrating her major books: *The Field, The Intention Experiment,* and *The Bond.*

Whereas fundamental science is an important cornerstone of a paradigm shift for curriculum, applied science is just as important. **Yury Kronn, PhD,** earned his post-doctorate degree at Russia's leading research institute and is world-renowned as a research scientist and inventor. Dr. Kronn was educated in the physics of nonlinear vibrations at some of the world's premier schools: Gorky University (former USSR) and Lebedev's Institute of Physics in Moscow. He has become one of the leading researchers in the application of the principles of quantum physics, developing a line of products and a network of connections to promote and advance the understanding of subtle energies. His contributions have been an inspiration for the university over the past ten years, and he continues to add important information to the design of new programs, supported by his innovative research in the field. Dr. Kronn has been a regular presenter at our World Congress of Quantum Medicine and, at the time of writing this, is developing a new course for Quantum University.

Bruce Lipton, PhD, also a featured presenter in the movie *What the Bleep Do We Know?!* has added to the curriculum of the university a new perspective regarding evolution in his course on the biology of belief (Lipton 2013).

Dr. Lipton is internationally recognized as a stem-cell biologist, a best-selling author of *The Biology of Belief* (2005), and recipient of the 2009 Goi Peace Award. Since 1982, he has been examining the principles of quantum physics and how they may be integrated into his understanding of the cell's information processing systems. He has produced breakthrough studies on the cell membrane, which revealed that this outer layer of the cell is an organic homologue of a computer chip, the cell's equivalent of a brain. His view on evolution was a perfect fit for quantum medicine and is very complementary to the tremendous work being done by Dr. Joe Dispenza.

Dr. Yury Kronn has recently joined our faculty to present another important aspect of the application of the principles of quantum physics to healing. Dr. Kronn is a world-renowned research scientist, inventor, theoretician, Human Rights activist and organizer, educated at one of the world's premier schools in the area of the physics of nonlinear vibrations, Gorky University (former USSR). He earned his post doctorate degree at Russia's leading research institute, Lebedev's Institute of Physics in Moscow and became one of the leading researchers and theoreticians heading up research on high frequency electromagnetic vibrations, laser physics and nonlinear optics. He was a lecturer and adjunct professor at the Physics and Technical Institute of Moscow University, where he taught bachelor and doctoral students a variety of courses in nonlinear optics, quantum electronics and quantum mechanics. Dr. Kronn is dedicated to researching and refining these applications, developing a line of products, and developing a network of connections to promote and advance the understanding of subtle energies.

Mind-Based Medicine

With **Patrick Porter, PhD,** joining the faculty, Quantum University was able to offer core knowledge regarding mind-based medicine. Dr. Porter has dedicated his life to empowering others through the use of the mind. He has twenty-four years of experience in the field of neurolinguistic programming (NLP) and hypnotherapy and teaches courses on both of these subjects at Quantum University. He is also the creator of our master's degree program in mind-based medicine. As part of this program, he has brought the renowned **Richard Bandler, PhD**, cofounder of neurolinguistic programming and author/coauthor of numerous books on NLP and its applications, to our team.

Dr. Porter is also an award-winning author of books, which include *Awaken the Genius: Mind Technology for the 21st Century* (1993), *Discover the Language of the Mind* (1994), *Six Secrets of G.E.N.I.U.S.* (1997), and *Thrive in Overdrive* (2009). He is the founder of the Positive Changes franchise network and the innovator of ZenFrames™/MindFit technologies, with which we codeveloped the Quantum Superlearning Technology for our students. Together with his wife, **Cynthia Porter, PhD**, they have also put together a quantum entrepreneur course (Porter) based on their years of successful franchise ownership.

Dr. Joe Dispenza's addition to the faculty reinforces an important piece of the curriculum regarding neuroscience with his course on the brain and neuroplasticity (2013). Joe Dispenza, DC, studied biochemistry at Rutgers University in New Brunswick, New Jersey, and also holds a BS degree with an emphasis in neuroscience. He received his doctor of chiropractic degree at Life University in Atlanta, Georgia, graduating magna cum laude. Dr. Dispenza has traveled to numerous countries throughout the world, conducting workshops and educating people on how to "reprogram their thinking through scientifically proven neuro-physiologic principles … founded in his total conviction that every person on this planet has within them the latent potential of greatness and true unlimited abilities."

Dr. Dispenza has certainly written a chapter that will make history in both quantum and modern medicine with his book and DVD *Evolve Your Brain: The Science of Changing Your Mind* (2007) and his books *Breaking the Habit of Being Yourself: How to Lose Your Mind and Create a New One* (2012), and *You Are the Placebo* (2014). His works and ongoing research based on the latest understandings of neuroscience will definitely be a part of the annals of medicine. A curriculum intending to illustrate a new paradigm for medicine based on quantum physics would have been incomplete without this masterpiece of understanding of the mechanics of the neurocircuity of the brain.

Seeing how we create new brain circuits in the brain that are the witness of a new reality imprint offers a growing awareness for clients who have been guided through quantum creativity or other experiences that generated quantum leaps. This is the practicality of a concept that would have been disregarded without scientific proof or a specific strategy to attempt to reproduce these extraordinary phenomena. In doing this, Dr. Dispenza is not alone.

Dr. Jeffrey L. Fannin holds a PhD in Psychology, an MBA and a BS degree in Mass Communications, and is the main designer of the neurofeedback certification program, a key program in our curriculum that will allow doctors and professional health practitioners to implement a new technology called Quantitative Electroencephalography (QEEG) in their clinics.

Dr. Fannin has worked in neuroscience for over 15 years and is the founder and executive director of the Center for Cognitive Enhancement. He has extensive experience training the brain for optimal performance, working with head trauma and recovery, stroke, chronic pain, Attention Deficit Disorder, anxiety disorders, and depression. His cutting-edge research uses electroencephalogram (EEG) technology to accurately measure balanced brainwave energy, which he has identified as the whole-brain state. This research focuses on subconscious belief patterns—translating limited personal success into balanced brain performance. His work as part of a team at Arizona State University researching neuroscience and leadership, including work at the United States Military Academy at West Point, led him to develop a course on "The Neuroscience of Leadership." His recent research pursues the effect of subtle energy in the quantum field and its effect on the brain.

Auriculotherapy

Dr. Terry Oleson's course on auriculotherapy is a unique, integral addition to our curriculum. Dr. Oleson, an internationally known leader in the field of auriculotherapy, has a PhD in psychobiology from the University of California at Irvine. In 1973, he conducted pioneering research on auricular diagnosis and auricular acupuncture at the UCLA Pain Management Center. He has authored numerous scientific articles and two books on auricular acupuncture, including the *Auriculotherapy Manual: Chinese and Western Systems of Ear Acupuncture* (1996) and the *International Handbook of Ear Reflex Points* (1997). Dr. Oleson is the research director at the American University of complementary medicine, chair of the Department of Psychology at the California Graduate Institute, and teacher here at Quantum University.

Aromatherapy

Another key area of study we wanted to incorporate into our curriculum was aromatherapy. **Debrah Zepf, PhD**, a board-certified master herbalist through the American Naturopathic Medical Certification Board, a certified bio-energetic practitioner and one of our graduate students in natural medicine, recently joined our faculty to develop and teach a course on aromatherapy for our students.

Natural and Integrative Medicine

Early on, **Dr. Faith Nelson**, a registered nurse with a PhD in integrative medicine, joined our team. With over twenty-eight years of experience and her broad expertise in allopathic medicine and critical care, as well as complementary alternative approaches within a variety of health-care settings, she has played a central role in creating the integrative Holistic Health Care Program here at Quantum University.

As a medical doctor, my own area of expertise has been to lay the clinical groundwork for integrating all of these aspects of our quantum physics-based curriculum together with other aspects of natural medicine into an applied clinical framework that can be used by our students as they develop their own approaches to treatment. Some of the content of these programs has been discussed in previous chapters of this book: evaluation, hematology, homeopathy, quantum Taoist medicine, hormonology, and quantum creativity.

We are grateful for the wealth of knowledge and experience brought together by our prestigious teachers and contributors, which continues to provide the essential building blocks for expressing a new model of health-care education based on an understanding of quantum physics. With the addition of new courses by Dr. Joe Dispenza, Dr. Jeffrey Fannin, Lynne McTaggart, and Dr. Yury Kronn, we are continuously working to grow our educational foundation to inspire a new generation of health-care practitioners. We are pleased to add these world-renowned personalities to an existing foundation of very respectable teachers who are articulating the essentials of a curriculum inspired by the new ideas of quantum physics and integrative medicine.

In Conclusion

As you have seen in this chapter, it takes a family to raise a child—some would say a village—but in this situation, a collective consciousness of renowned scientists.

How we can teach outdated information in medical universities for so many years is very disappointing and sad. The weak and the sick are locked into an unaffordable health-care system currently limited in its capacity to offer all possibilities for healing.

Can you imagine that, thirty years ago, the type of discussion we are having today would have been completely irrelevant? Of course, great minds and renowned scientists have been master players in bringing this knowledge forward, but without a collective awareness to make possible the manifestation of new ways of healing, this would be impossible.

The notable information brought by our prestigious teachers is essential as building blocks to express a model of health-care education representing the new paradigm shift as defined by quantum physics. But how to draw these new principles on the clinical ground has been my task and area of expertise.

The major goal has been to spin out what is taught. I recognized that a more conventional naturopathy, or natural medicine out of a mold, is repeating the same old model of thinking as does conventional medicine. Replacing pharmaceuticals with natural products may quiet your mind, but it will not make that much of a difference if your model of healing is not expanded according to a greater experience of reality.

What really matters is to finally look at the human being in terms of infinite possibilities, whereby a means to restore health could be also infinite. These new notions of perceiving a broader reality must be laid out in a curriculum that will not only reflect them but also practically implement them in a clinical manner. A program is ever definitive and should continue to be improved as our understanding is deepened.

Chapter 8
Creative Integrative Medical Solutions for Health Care

Einstein said, "We cannot solve our problems with the same thinking we used when we created them." Coming from a background of experience with both social and privatized health-care systems, I am convinced that simply adjusting socio-political methods for delivery is not enough to solve the current health-care crisis.

One of the most important phenomena on my journey to evolve from a linear medical model to a multidimensional model of healing was not just to broaden my toolbox with extra modalities of healing, but to radically transform my relationship with the client from one where I was caught in a fatalistic perspective (diagnostic) with no other outcome in addressing the symptoms to one of a greater awareness. This made possible many results—from spontaneous remissions to personal growth—within an environment that acknowledged the objectivity as well as the subjectivity of the experience.

Medical health care needs first to be reformed at its base, as the real cost of healing is directly associated with how healing is practiced in this society. What I mean by its base is by how doctors and health-care practitioners are initially trained and educated regarding the art of healing.

Why this issue is not at the top of our conversation at such a critical moment, where everything is on the verge of completely falling apart, can only be understood if we start to investigate the conflicts of interest related to it.

But before we get into this issue, I would like to suggest to you a simple exercise that I will call "Imagine."

America is the perfect arena for such an exercise.

Imagine that the founding fathers of this great country couldn't perceive of the possibility of a greater country.

Imagine that Abraham Lincoln, in the midst of the Civil War, couldn't intuit the possible freedom associated with slavery at that time.

Imagine that most of the great inventors couldn't have seen that planes could fly, sound could travel through space, electricity could be conducted through a wire …

Imagine that doctors, nurses, and health-care practitioners in this society didn't have access to *the field* as a source of all healing in the art of healing.

Imagine doctors, nurses, and health-care practitioners in this society being trapped in a limited model of medicine that didn't believe that the impossible could happen—spontaneous remissions.

Imagine doctors, nurses, and health-care practitioners in this society blinded by .0000001 percent of reality (dark matter) and unable to see the subtle energy anatomy of the individual.

Imagine doctors, nurses, and health-care practitioners in this society themselves separated from the experience of healing, unaware of their healing entanglement with the client.

Imagine that the most precious information regarding healing is completely absent from our medical curriculum and that great doctors and health-care practitioners in this society can't understand the mechanics of mind, body, spirit.

This list can go on and on, but I am sure you already feel the constraints, limitations, and tremendous costs that are linked to a rationale associated with an outdated model of science that is no longer adequate in our modern time.

Let's see what could be implemented with creativity. The complexity of the health-care crisis will require innovative solutions if it is to be solved. The politico-social approach is a component of this solution, but obviously, as we said, insufficient. The costs related to conventional medical approaches, which are disease-oriented and limited to surgery and pharmaceutical therapies, is out of reach of the wallet of many societies, rich or poor, as we have discussed in previous chapters.

Before elaborating on some concrete strategies that can make a difference and release the tremendous financial pressure that we are facing at this time in America, let's review some major points that we have presented so far.

1. Conventional and natural medicine education must be redefined on the premise of an updated model of science based on the principles of quantum physics.

2. New and ancient models of healing must be available through the health-care system as possibilities of healing when they meet the requirements of this new model of science. It doesn't mean that everything should get a pass simply because it is labeled "quantum." We must exercise the same rigor of science but with an enlarged foundation of understanding.

3. We need an approach to medicine that is health-oriented, seeking the full potential of the individual, instead of a fatalistic disease perspective of the individual.

4. A new paradigm shift, to be credible, must be defined by doctors and teachers who have been able to, in this modern time, impress a worldwide scientific community through their publications and research.

5. The humanitarian component of this new medicine must be developed with sensitivity to the needs of our communities.

A positive approach to this health-care crisis will be to propose what I call Health-Care Management: Creative Integrative Medicine. What I am proposing is to incorporate into the health-care system a radical view for implementing modalities of healing with a deeper understanding of the reality of healing as revealed by an updated model of medical science, as defined by quantum physics.

The Economics of Health Care

Again, back to Einstein's quote: "We cannot solve our problems with the same thinking we used when we created them." This implies training and education. When we bring forth the subject of education today, we become involved automatically in another painful fact.

"Student debt burden hits $1 trillion." (Herships 2012).

"Some students (medical) are graduating with more than $200,000 in debt" (Hopkins 2011).

This is why the delivery of essential information must cost less. The lowered cost of education should immediately result in decreased health-care costs and new revenue streams for the doctors and practitioners who become trained in creative integrative medicine. I refer you to the previous chapter to understand that the future of education, in terms of effectiveness and profitability, must include delivery through high-tech online technology.

Having been involved in the setup of many medical environments myself—from an ER, to a preventative and medical family clinic, to a hospital—I have a precise understanding that doctors, nurses, and other health-care practitioners are already overwhelmed by their regular tasks. Not only that, but doctors have seen their earnings decreasing, considering they have increasingly more bureaucratic functions to do.

This reality is substantiated in a 2008 report by the Medical Group Management Association.

> Compounding economic pressures created by declining reimbursement and crushing administrative burdens, operating costs rose faster than revenue in many medical group practices in 2007, according to the Medical Group Management Association (MGMA) Cost Survey: 2008 Reports Based on 2007 Data. MGMA data indicate that over the past decade, operating expenses have risen from 58 cents to 61 cents per dollar of revenue.
>
> Multispecialty group practices reported a 5.5 percent increase in median total revenue; median operating costs increased by 6.5 percent (MGMA 2008).

How can this equation be solved? On one side, we are talking about adding more work to a health-care team that is already overwhelmed by their tasks. On the other side, if you look more closely at the whole portrait of the health-care business, there is a new phenomenon emerging in the health-care industry.

> Even in these recessionary times, a great deal of money is being spent on some forms of complementary and alternative medicine ..." said Bruce Silverglade, director of legal affairs for the Center for Science in the Public Interest, a consumer advocacy group ... The average annual spending per person to see practitioners was about $122, and the average spending on products was $177 Associated Press 2009).

Other sources of information confirm the same trend in the health-care industry.

A report by Jason Luban in August 2011 stated,

> The most recent study of CAM usage I could find was in the New England Journal of Medicine (NEJM) from 1997. It showed that the number of Americans using an alternative therapy rose from 33% in 1990 to 42% in 1997, and some research estimates that the number may be as high as 70% today. The NEJM study also found that, in 1997, Americans spent more than $27 billion on these therapies, exceeding out-of-pocket spending for all US hospitalizations, and that the number of patient visits to CAM providers exceeded those to primary care physicians (Luban 2011).

At this time, the health-care system seems completely dormant regarding this new need and demand from the society. More than that, natural medicine is often looked down upon and ridiculed by an argument that doesn't hold anymore: "This is not scientific." Instead of being a part of it and remodeling the image of health care with approaches that are more natural and with fewer side effects, the tendency is to align with pharmaceutical companies that no longer have the favor of the public. This situation can be changed overnight by the comprehensive type of approach that is being proposed in this book.

Another very important piece of information that we must add to this analysis is to have the capacity to be able to change the equation.

Cash Practice Alternatives: Considerations for Physicians
Physicians seeking ways to simplify their practices and reduce administrative overhead are evaluating whether limiting their financial dependence on health insurer

contracts is a viable option. Many of these physicians are turning to an array of alternatives often referred to as "cash practices (AMA Practice Management Center 2008).

To reiterate the whole problematic situation, we have on one hand a health-care industry that has a desperate need to refresh its strategies for healing to make it more efficient and affordable, and on the other hand, a huge market for alternative or integrative natural medicine. In the middle are overworked and underpaid health-care staff seeking an approach to health care that is more rewarding and professionally gratifying. The issue of having more rewarding work is also an important factor affecting the recovery of the client/patient. Even though the National Institute of Health's NCBI-US National Library of Medicine has recognized nursing as "the most emotionally rewarding career" (Waters 2008), we have seen many overworked health-care practitioners looking for other careers due to the pressures of the milieu.

Proposals for Integration of This New Model into the Existing Health-Care System

Implementing an integrative medicine solution with a new awareness of healing would, at this juncture, add to a health-care practitioner's multiple levels of training. These additional abilities and modalities could then be the source of new income for a family clinic or other medical service environment.

Expand Training and Roles of Medical Assistants and Nurses

The medical assistant is already doing basic work for the doctor in medical clinics. Being trained professionally with a basic understanding of these new modalities, medical assistants could become key players by assisting the doctor and helping to offer services that the clients are already seeking in the community, currently without professional supervision.

A medical assistant could be trained as a holistic medical assistant and be the one who begins implementation of basic protocols for weight loss, smoking cessation, pain management, insomnia, anxiety, or attention deficit hyperactivity disorder (to name a few), under the supervision of the medical doctor.

The long-term consequence of earlier protocols being implemented into the patient's health-care plan could also have the effect of decreasing the costs associated with debilitating and chronic diseases. The doctor would have more satisfaction in doing his work and would be able to respond to the need to take good care of his/her clientele by addressing the root cause of their health issues.

Nurses and medical assistants could upgrade their credentials and abilities by pursuing bachelor's, master's, and doctorate degrees in integrative medicine. Building on the foundation of their previous education, they would only have to add the complementary components to their education to give them the understanding of the principles of this new medicine and also the capacity to implement more complex modalities.

Educate the Health-Care Administrators and Decision Makers

I am always shocked to see that the management of health care is handled by administrators who have had very little training or knowledge in the art of healing. I remember that when they began to implement social medicine in Canada, major decisions were being made by administrators who had no idea about health care and healing. Education in integrative medicine should also be introduced to this community of decision makers as part of the strategy of reallocation of resources, providing them with a broader perspective and the ability to make better choices. In quantum physics, everything is about perception of reality. How different would our decisions be if they were based upon multiple possibilities of choice and empowered by creativity?

Offer a Specialty in Integrative Medicine for Medical Doctors

Finally, one of the major players is the medical doctor. These members of the health-care team are already looking for a specialty in integrative medicine.

The two major difficulties that a physician faces are the time factor in getting trained and how they will be able to implement these new modalities when they are already overburdened by their regular tasks. I think we already have an answer to these two questions. If I, as a medical doctor in the midst of a busy practice, found the time to study acupuncture, homeopathy, and naturopathy, how can a medical doctor with the support of online and iPad technology not do more?

At our university, we have already graduated many medical doctors who have become engaged with this path. To answer the other aspect of the question, you must understand that the physician will need to be surrounded by a team of health-care practitioners that have also been trained within the same framework and who will be implementing the protocols and modalities that he or she doesn't have the time to do personally. Again, keep in mind that family clinics and medical centers will be offering services that will generate new income, with the satisfaction that the clientele is taken care of at the root of their health issues. This will create a win-win situation for the health-care system, the client, and for the team of health-care practitioners who will feel more rewarded for their dedicated work.

Change from a Doctor-Centered to Patient-Empowered Approach

Another important component of this global strategy is to decentralize the health-care system, which is currently centered on the doctor. Instead, we must create a system centered on the individual patient/client who can be educated by a group of health-care practitioners trained in this new understanding of integrative medicine.

Two of the beliefs of Quantum University are that "everyone should be educated on how to heal themselves and others" and "the right to heal belongs to everyone who sincerely manifests and desires it" (IQUIM, Mission and Belief Statements).

Of course, the health-care system plays an important role in the health of the individual, but being empowered to be healthy should not be based on the belief that the health-care system is the only omnipotent source of healing.

This new perspective of the reality and responsibility for healing should be known by everybody, and the knowledge of it should be the focus of our society. Ignorance has a very high cost, which can be exploited by all the conflicts of interest associated with the health industry. Isn't knowledge the beginning of freedom?

One of the most virulent debates in the next decades will be on the subject of prevention, genetics, and the role of pharmaceuticals and surgery in changing the trajectory of a predictable disease. A model of education based on the biology of possibilities—where the genes are not the only determinant factor in the equation concerning the genesis of diseases, but where our own perceptions and beliefs are recognized as being just as important in the outcome of our health—will have enormous economic and social consequences for health care. A model of education that is more refined in the understanding of the subtle energies and the connection between mind and body will have more consequence in the resolution of chronic diseases and cancer than any heavy medical approaches at this time. Brain plasticity and neuroscience are already changing all the parameters of the dinosaurian views taught at medical universities.

After a second look at the history of medicine, everyone comes to recognize the evidence that hygiene has contributed more to the regression of infections in hospitals than the advent of antibiotics. One day, we will come to a similar conclusion that knowledge based on a more accurate and scientific perception, when integrated into a model of medical education, will do more to contribute to our population being not only healthier but also living longer than within our existing system.

How do you feel when you are exposed every day to pharmaceutical TV advertisements that try to sell you a pill to take for a disease more serious than the side effects associated with the medication? Obviously, shouldn't you choose the least harmful choice between the two catastrophes?

In order to empower people's health care, these new quantum paradigms in science must be included in university curricula for both traditional medicine and natural medicine, as well as taught to the general public. Doctors and health-care providers need to be educated through this updated model of science. The responsibility for health should not depend solely on the medical health-care system but on educating the public in this new, empowering concept of achieving full potential in health. By finding a way to integrate both natural and conventional medicine under a new integrative health-care system, in conjunction with the wellness industry, society's health care will be best served.

Chapter 9
Conclusion

Quantum physics teaches us that we are the makers of our own reality.

In this book, I have revealed the personal journey that brought me to what I call today creative integrative medicine. When I look back over these years, I recognize that it has all emerged from within, triggered by the tragic death of my own brother. This personal journey has been an enlightening process that has allowed me to become more whole and integrated in my life.

I have kept for the end the story of a strange and at the same time fabulous dream I had when I was twenty-two years old. There were two parts to this dream that I couldn't explain in detail until I saw them within this current context. The first part gave me insight into what was coming in my life, including my debate with the medical world. The second was a profound spiritual revelation that one day I hope I can dedicate another book to. This dream brought me to an experience almost impossible to describe in words, and I would like at least to reveal my immediate impression when I woke up.

On CNN in 2013, as part of the *Anderson Cooper Special Report: To Heaven and Back*, incredible stories about individuals sharing near-death experiences were presented. I don't want to get into a theological debate as to whether these individuals really did die and come back

145

from heaven. My point is more about their transcendent experience of a luminous and bright reality or expansion of awareness, about how after they came back to their usual state of mind, things didn't look the same any more.

Dr. Deepak Chopra, in *Quantum Healing* (1989), describes quantum leaps of awareness that, in the definitive, make spontaneous healing happen. In Anderson Cooper's special report, Anita Moorjani, in her final moments with stage 4 lymphoma cancer, realized through an extraordinary experience of unconditional love that there was no longer a reason to fear and nurture her cancer. Within a few months, her cancer totally disappeared, even though her doctors couldn't understand why.

Dr. Goswami has also described how the supramental, through intuition, can manifest spontaneous healing (as discussed in chapter 2 on quantum creativity). The context of the experience doesn't really matter: a near-death experience, a dream, a moment of clarity under a tree (Newton), or in your bath (Archimedes). What really matters is that something profound has changed forever in your experience of reality. Envisioning something that doesn't belong to the linear perception of your senses will transform you forever. This is the type of impression that I had when I woke up that morning in the winter of 1972. An *au de la* experience that would change my life in ways that I could not even understand at that time.

How can a dream prepare you or at least inform you about what has not yet happened? Quantum physics has an explanation for how time isn't exactly what our linear-focused mind thinks it is. I am not the first one who has had premonitions. There are many such phenomena described in literature; however, it took years before I could put all the pieces together and understand the full meaning of the dream. But as the stream of my life has been unfolding, I have begun to understand my participation in a play which is greater than I am, where at the same time destiny and freedom intertwine, as do the dichotomies of reality of wave and particle in the quantum world.

In writing this book, my intent was also for you to witness a process of awakening, where I progressively opened myself to new knowledge and possibilities for healing. In the beginning, this was an imperceptible seed, a veil, dormant in my inner self. I couldn't see exactly where it was going. I let myself go with the flow (sometimes with resistance), and after thirty years, I have just begun to see where this adventure is heading.

I realize that I am taking a risk by sharing this information at the end of the book. Some readers may question whether I'm a little crazy. But I decided to take the risk because I am not the only one who has experienced these phenomena. Unusual experiences are far more common that we can imagine, and altered states of consciousness happening naturally are being described more and more often.

In 1978–1979, when I went to Switzerland and studied with an advanced group of meditators (also medical doctors), we were already investigating altered states of consciousness using EEGs. Today, neuroscience has refined its technology for what we call brain mapping. Last summer, in the context of Dr. Joe Dispenza's workshop, I had the opportunity to have a brain map done on myself while I was going into a particular state of meditation. It was an amazing experience to have neuro-feedback of an inner-world experience, where my mind was actively integrating information. The results of this experiment were presented at our last World Congress of Quantum Medicine in 2013. You can also find more information about it at http://iquim.org/quantum-world-tv/paul-drouin/world-congress-2013-highlights/ (IQUIM, World Congress 2013 Highlights).

The brain-map results revealed a high degree of neuroplasticity and that I was able to integrate both logical and intuitive information at the same time. I also had the capacity to maintain a state of meditation for more than the usual amount of time. As I was in a bliss state during most of the experience, the results showed many gamma waves with a high state of coherence. I am sharing this information not to be pretentious but to demonstrate that my mind seems to work perfectly well, like many others who see a little more of the world than .0000001 percent of reality.

Today, I can say that for me, medicine has been a path of personal growth, integration, and discovery that has allowed me to express my compassion and love for the world. I consider this to be a very great privilege and believe that healing with awareness is certainly the most beautiful thing to experience. The same thing is happening in our society. Ideas and concepts are evolving. Thirty years ago, when I published a review of literature on transcendental meditation with another group of doctors, nobody understood what its relationship with medicine was. A journalist wrote in a local journal, "This funny doctor …" Today, there are many doctors who recommend to their patients to relax and sign up for yoga or meditation classes.

When I previously wrote in the journal *Medecin du Québec* on the controversial subject of yeast syndrome and timidly suggested that an antibiotic regimen should be followed up by a preventive intake of probiotics to balance the bowel flora, this upset the whole community of infectologists in Québec. They subsequently presented an article denying the problem in the following month. Now this is a common prescription that is suggested by a pharmacist, if the doctor doesn't recommend it, to avoid frequent complications from antibiotics.

In other words, society is heading in the same direction today as I did, even though it is with resistance and all sorts of conflicts of interest. This movement is inevitable because it is toward the truth, and it is common sense to evolve toward more possibilities for health and well-being for the common good. Being healthy is inherent to the pursuit of happiness and is a right dear to the American people. How is this right being respected if in our modern society health and the ability to realize the full potential of the individual are not available to everyone? The only solution is to welcome more creativity and intelligence into the way we generate and sustain these rights.

In the midst of my fight for natural medicine, one of the main arguments—that these modalities or means of investigation can't be used to help a patient, even when all other conventional medical resources have been exhausted—is no longer sustainable. Now these new concepts of healing, as demonstrated in this book, can be sustained by the quantum physics model of science and be taught in universities—as they are at Quantum University. The new emerging neuroscience is also moving in this direction.

There was a time when it was convenient to think that the earth was flat, but then came a time when reality could no longer be denied. It is the same in medicine. There was a time when it was convenient to believe in a materialistic point of view of human health, but reality cannot be denied anymore!

Modern medicine is in crisis. Somewhere along the way, it lost its soul as its roots grew into a materialistic foundation that acknowledges only an infinitesimal part of reality. The tree of medicine must be transplanted into new soil, where its roots can deepen and intertwine to reach a more complex source of healing knowledge and bring together all traditions of healing, ancient and modern.

I envision that modern medicine will have no choice but to take this path. On one hand, the economic and financial pressures on the health-care system show it is no longer affordable. On the other hand, there is the growing awareness of a collective consciousness that is experiencing a new level of reality through a growing understanding of quantum medicine.

Quantum University has allowed me to discover a large community of people from all over the world who have come to hold a similar vision for healing through many avenues of growth. Collective consciousness is intertwining with individual awareness that is creating a butterfly effect in the medical world!

I can now envision, merging from all directions, a new generation of healers and doctors trained in the creative integrative medicine vision, based on the foundation of quantum physics and applied to a deeper understanding of human beings.

This will enable us to tap into infinite fields of healing because modern medicine will have broadened the frontiers of the perception of the human reality. This is why it is so important to establish a new model of science in the current system of medical education, just as we are doing at Quantum University.

Thirty years ago, my colleagues would smile when the subject of alternative medicine was brought forward, but not anymore. The old concepts now seem out-of-date and my old colleagues are ready to retire, whereas students educated in these new concepts of spontaneous healing are ready to challenge health care with more intelligence and creativity.

In the coming decades, this new foundation of understanding of the human being will open up infinitely greater numbers of applications for healing. When we look back at how we have limited our resources to pharmaceuticals and surgery in the last century, we will not only be disappointed in a system of medicine that too closely resembles that of the Middle Ages, we will be embarrassed that it took us so long to realize that the real debate must focus on how medicine is practiced. We must make sure that the premises of healing don't continue to be based on such a narrow-minded point of view!

A Future Vision for Health Care

This is a very exciting time to be alive. Out of what we feel could be a medical catastrophe will emerge a more creative and humanistic way to become whole again. How the new health care will look in the next twenty years is out of reach of a linear model of thinking. Emergency medicine will also evolve with more specialized care as expected, but the core foundation of health will be recentered around the reality of the full potential of the individual, instead of disease. The individual will be able to reappropriate the right to heal through costless and affordable technologies available to everyone on the planet.

Knowledge of health, through a renaissance in medical education, will open resources for healing that will make what we are doing now look like it's from another age. The evaluation of the client, that I provided some premise for in a previous chapter, will be supported by a technology much more refined than we now know—a technology with fewer side effects and with the capacity to access subtle energy and identify disease at an earlier stage where dramatic interventions can be avoid. Preventive care will be shared with clients equipped with friendly technologies that can support a positive life style and decrease traffic in the clinics. Going to the hospital will be a last resort after all other means of therapies have been exhausted—prevention and family clinics being first and second—except, of course, in the case of emergencies.

The repertory of therapies will be universal, giving access to many traditions of healing, as long as they can be supported by the new science of quantum physics applied to healing. Hospitals and clinics will be well equipped with complementary care and competent health-care practitioners trained in integrative medicine.

We are not far from this vision. The trigger for this health-care revolution will be a renaissance in medical education, as the concepts of *Creative Integrative Medicine,* such as those that I have presented in this book, continue to be implemented.

Works Cited

AMA Practice Management Center. "Cash Practice Alternatives: Considerations for Physicians." *Yumpu.* Jaunary 2, 2008. http://www.yumpu.com/en/document/view/11607436/cash-practice-alternatives-considerations-for-physicians-american-.

Associated Press (AP). "$34 Billion Spent Yearly on Alternative Medicine." *Alternative Medicine on NBCNews.com.* July 30, 2009. http://www.nbcnews.com/id/32219873/ns/health-alternative_medicine/#.Uw6hU4Wblss.

Blackburn, Diane. *Application of Quantum Medicine in Live Blood Analysis.* Unpublished doctoral dissertation, International Quantum University for Integrative Medicine (Quantum University), Honolulu, HI, 2013.

Blicher, B., F. Blondeau, C. Choquette, A. Deans, P. Drouin, J. Glaser, and P. Thibaudeau. "Méditation Transcendantale: Revue de la Littérature Scientifique." *Le Médecin du Québec* 15(8):46-66, 1980.

Bradford, Robert W. and Henry W. Allen. *Oxidology, The Study of Reactive Oxygen Species (Ros) and Their Metabolism in Health and Disease.* N.p.: Bradford Foundation, 1997.

Burns, C.P.E. "Wolfgang Pauli, Carl Jung, and the Acausal Connecting Principle: A Case Study in Transdisciplinarity." metanexus.net. September 1, 2011. http://www.metanexus.net/essay/wolfgang-pauli-carl-jung-and-acausal-connecting-principle-case-study-transdisciplinarity.

Cady, Roger K. and Norman Shealy. *Neurochemical Responses to Cranial Electrical Stimulation and Photo-Stimulation Via Brain Wave Synchronization*. Springfield, MO: Shealy Institute of Comprehensive Health Care, 1990.

Capra, Fritjof. *The Tao of Physics*. Boulder, CO: Shambhala, 1975.

Chopra, Deepak. *Quantum Healing: Exploring the Frontiers of Mind/Body Medicine*. New York: Bantam Books, 1989.

CNN - Anderson Cooper 360. "Anderson Cooper Special Report: To Heaven and Back." December 1, 2013. http://ac360.blogs.cnn.com/2013/11/27/anderson-cooper-special-report-to-heaven-and-back/.

Conarroe, Teresa. *Terry Conarroe*. International Quantum University for Integrative Medicine (Quantum University), n.d. http://iquim.org/testimonial-post/terry-conarroe/.

de Surany, Marguerite. *Dictionnaire de Medecine Taoist*. Montreal, Québec: Diffusion Edition Internationale, 376, avenue Lautrier Ouest, 1996.

— *le Corps d'Arc en Ciel (The Rainbow Body)*. Paris: Guy Tredaniel, Editeur, 65 rue Claude Bernard, Paris, 1996.

Dispenza, Joe. *Brain and Neuroplasticity Course*. International Quantum University for Integrative Medicine (Quantum University), May 2013. https://iquim.org/courses/brain-and-neuroplasticity/?n=ws&c=sta.

— *Breaking the Habit of Being Yourself: How to Lose Your Mind and Create a New One*. New York: Hay House, Inc., 2012.

— *Evolve Your Brain: The Science of Changing Your Mind*. Deerfield Beach, FL: Health Communications, Inc., 2007.

— *You Are the Placebo*. New York: Hay House, 2014.

Drouin, Paul. "Conference Tour "Seeing is Believing" - How Quantum Medicine Works in the Physical Body." International Quantum University for Integrative Medicine (Quantum University): Quantum World TV, 2009-2011. http://iquim.org/quantum-world-tv/paul-drouin/seeing-is-believing-quantum-medicine/.

— *Five Pillars of Health Course.* International Quantum University for Integrative Medicine (Quantum University), n.d. http://store.iquim.org/index.php?main_page=product_info&cPath=63&products_id=42.

— *Quantum Hematology Course.* International Quantum University for Integrative Medicine (Quantum University), n.d. http://store.iquim.org/index.php?main_page=product_info&cPath=63&products_id=40.

— *Quantum Hormonology Course.* International Quantum University for Integrative Medicine (Quantum University), n.d. http://store.iquim.org/index.php?main_page=product_info&cPath=63&products_id=43.

— *Quantum Taoist Medicine and Acupuncture Course.* International Quantum University for Integrative Medicine (Quantum University), n.d. http://store.iquim.org/index.php?main_page=product_info&products_id=44.

Emoto, Masaru. *The Hidden Messges in Water.* Hillsboro, OR: Beyond Words Publishing, Inc., 2001.

Enderlein, Günther. *Bacteria Cyclogeny: Prolegomena to a Study of the Structure, Sexual and Asexual Reproduction and Development of Bacteria.* Glendale, AZ: PleomorphicSANUM, 1925.

Feiler, Bruce. *Council of Dads,* n.d. http://councilofdads.ning.com/.

— *The Council of Dads: My Daughters, My Illness, and the Men Who Could Be Me.* New York: HarperCollins Publishers, 2010.

Gerber, Richard. *Vibrational Medicine: New Choices for Healing Ourselves.* Santa Fe, NM: Bear & Company, 1988.

Goswami, Amit. *God Is Not Dead: What Quantum Physics Tells Us about Our Origins And How We Should Live.* Charlottesville, VA: Hampton Roads Publishing Company, Inc., 2008.

— *Physics of the Soul: The Quantum Book of Living, Dying, Reincarnation and Immortality.* Charlottesville, VA: Hampton Roads Publishing Company, Inc., 2001.

— *Quantum Creativity: Think Quantum, Be Creative.* New York: Hay House, Inc., 2014.

— *Quantum Doctor Course.* International Quantum University for Integrative Medicine (Quantum University), n.d. http://store. iquim.org/index.php?main_page=product_info&cPath=86& products_id=126&zenid=jcsgg1ttl9sqla5ig7j6lqr885.

— *Quantum Mechanics.* Dubuque, IA: William C. Brown Publ., 1991.

— *The Physicists' View of Nature, Part 1: From Newton to Einstein.* New York: Kluwer Academic / Plenum Publishers, 2000.

— *The Physicists' View of Nature, Part 2: The Quantum Revolution.* New York: Kluwer Academic / Plenum Publishers, 2001.

— *The Quantum Doctor, A Physicist's Guide to Health and Healing.* Charlottesville, VA: Hampton Roads Publishing Company, Inc., 2004.

— *The Visionary Window: A Quantum Physicist's Guide to Enlightenment.* Wheaton, Il: Quest Books / The Theosophical Publishing House, 2006.

Goswami, Amit, with Richard E. Reed and Maggie Goswami. *The Self-Aware Universe: How Consciousness Creates the Material World.* New York: Jeremy P. Tarcher / Putnam, 1993.

Gupta, Sanjay. *Paging Dr. Gupta! See Sanjay's Special on THE COUNCIL OF DADS.* May 3, 2010. http://brucefeiler.com/2010/05/paging-dr-gupta-see-sanjays-special-on-the-council-of-dads/.

Hahnemann, Samuel. *The Organon of the Healing Art.* Dublin: W. F. Wakeman, 1833.

Hartman, Franz. *The Life and the Doctrines of Philippus Theophrastus, Bombast of Hohenheim Known by the Name of Paracelsus, 2nd Edition.* London and Edinburgh: Morrison and Gibs, Ltd, 1896.

Herships, Sally. "Student Debt Burden Hits $1 Trillion." *American Public Media - Marketplace - Education.* April 25, 2012. http://www.marketplace.org/topics/life/education/student.

Hopkins, Katy. "10 Medical Schools That Lead to Most Debt." *Yahoo News - US News & World Report.* April 14, 2011. http://www.usnews.com/education/best-graduate.

Institute of Education Sciences. "The Condition of Education 2010." *National Center for Education Statistics, US Dept of Education,* May, 2010. http://nces.ed.gov/pubs2010/2010028.pdf.

IQUIM. *Mission and Belief Statements,* International Quantum University for Integrative Medicine (Quantum University), n.d. http://iquim.org/about/mission-belief-statements/.

— *Quantum World TV,* International Quantum University for Integrative Medicine (Quantum University), n.d. http://iquim.org/quantum-world-tv/.

— "What is a Quantum Hero?" International Quantum University for Integrative Medicine (Quantum University), n.d. http://iquim.org/what-is-a-quantum-hero/#.

— "World Congress 2013 Highlights." International Quantum University for Integrative Medicine (Quantum University): Quantum World TV, n.d. http://iquim.org/quantum-world-tv/paul-drouin/world-congress-2013-highlights/.

K-PAX. DVD. Directed by Iain Softley. Los Angeles: Universal Studios, 2010.

Knox, Patricia. "A True Quantum Hero and Autism." International Quantum University for Integrative Medicine (Quantum University): Quantum World TV, n.d. http://iquim.org/quantum-world-tv/paul-drouin/true-quantum-hero-autism/.

Lipton, Bruce H. *Biology of Belief Course.* International Quantum University for Integrative Medicine (Quantum University), May, 2013. http://store.iquim.org/index.php?main_page=product_info&products_id=34.

— *The Biology of Belief: Unleashing the Power of Consciousness, Matter and Miracles.* New York: Hay House, Inc, 2007.

Luban, Jason. "Toward a New Definition of Health." *PracticeRapport.com.* August 8, 2011. http://www.practicerapport.com/toward-a-new-definition-of-health-2.

Marcus, Suzanna. *6 Months to Live 10 Years Later: An Extraordinary Healing Journey.* Open Doorways Press, 2007.

McTaggart, Lynne. *Field Trilogy Masterclass.* International Quantum University for Integrative Medicine (Quantum University), n.d. https://iquim.org/courses/the-field-trilogy/.

— *The Bond: How to Fix Your Falling-Down World.* New York: Free Press / Simon & Schuster, Inc., 2011.

— *The Field: The Quest for the Secret Force of the Universe.* New York: HarperCollins Publishers, 2008.

— *The Intention Experiment: Using Your Thoughts to Change Your Life and the World.* New York: Free Press / Simon & Schuster, Inc., 2007.

— *What Doctors Don't Tell You: The Truth about the Dangers of Modern Medicine.* New York: Avon Books, 1996.

MGMA, Press Room. "Medical group-practice cost increases outpace revenues." *MGMA - Medical Group Management Association.* Oct 20, 2008. http://www.mgma.com/press/default.aspx?id=22678.

Oleson, Terry. *Auriculotherapy Manual: Chinese and Western Systems of Ear Acupuncture.* N.p.: Health Care Alternatives, 1996.

— *International Handbook of Ear Reflex Points.* N.p.: Health Care Alternatives, 1997.

Pascal, Blaise. *Pensées.* Paris: Guillaume Desprez, 1669.

Porter, Patrick K. *Awaken the Genius: Mind Technology for the 21st Century.* N.p.: Pure Light Publications, 1993.

— *Discover the Language of the Mind.* N.p.: PorterVision, LLC., 1994.

— *Thrive in Overdrive: How to Navigate Your Overloaded Lifestyle.* N.p.: PorterVision, LLC., 1994.

Porter, Patrick K., and Cynthia Porter. *Quantum Entrepreneur Course,* International Quantum University for Integrative Medicine (Quantum University), n.d. http://store.iquim.org/index.php?main_page=index&cPath=64.

— *Six Secrets of G.E.N.I.U.S.* New Bern, NC: Brain Wellness Unlimited, 1997.

Rudell, Wendy. *Dr. Wendy Rudell - June 19th, 2010.* International Quantum University for Integrative Medicine (Quantum University): Quantum World TV, 2010. http://iquim.org/quantum-world-tv/wendy-rudell/june-19-2010/.

Swartz, Kimberly. "Health cXre Xost Monitor." thehastingscenter. org. January 22, 2010. http://healthcarecostmonitor. thehastingscenter.org/kimberlyswartz/ projected-costs-of-chronic-diseases/.

The Living Matrix - The New Science of Healing. DVD. Directed by Greg Becker and Harry Massey. San Francisco: Beyond Words Pub., 2009.

Toufexis, Anastasia. "Is Homeopathy Good Medicine?" Time.com, September 25, 1995. http://content.time.com/time/magazine/ article/0,9171,983466,00.html.

Waters, A. "Nursing Is the Most Emotionally Rewarding Career" [From: Nurs Stand., 19(30):22-6]. *PubMed.gov.* April 6-12, 2005. http://www.ncbi.nlm.nih.gov/pubmed/15835432.

What the Bleep Do We Know!? DVD. Directed by William Arntz, Betsy Chasse, and Mark Vicente. Los Angeles: 20th Century Fox, 2004.

Wikipedia. "Pay It Forward." wikipedia.com, n.d. http://en.wikipedia. org/wiki/Pay_it_forward.

— "Pierre Teilhard de Chardin." wikipedia.org, n.d. http:// en.wikipedia.org/wiki/Pierre_Teilhard_de_Chardin.